MW00398660

Body Under Construction

How to Build and Maintain
Optimal Health at 20, 30, or 40+

TO

Jim Life Abundantly

(1 Samuel 25:6 ; 3 John 2)

Copyright 2011 Sloan J. Luckie
All rights reserved.

ISBN: 1460938895
ISBN 13: 9781460938898

Body Under Construction

Body Under Construction

How to Build and Maintain Optimal Health at 20, 30, or 40+

BY SLOAN J. LUCKIE

"It is never too late to be what you might have been"

- George Eliot

Contents

Preface: "Under Construction" · xiii

Introduction: Building and Maintaining Optimal Health · xv

Chapter One: Getting Started · 1

Chapter Two: Build and Maintain Optimal Health Through Optimal Nutrition · · · · · · · · · · · · · · · 3
   Eating Like a Teenager · 3
   Read the Label and Avoid THE 7 · 4
   A Smooth Start · 6
   Add Cereal to Your Fruit · 9
   "Let's Do Lunch": The Healthy Way · 11
   Dinner: The Most Dangerous Meal of the Day · 19
   And for Dessert... · 26
   Danger Zone (DZ) Snacks · 27

Chapter Three: Build and Maintain Optimal Health Through Optimal Fitness · · · · · · · · · · 31
   A Fitness Adventure · 31
   Pre-Fitness Adventure Tips · 32
   Day One and Day Two Fitness Adventure · 34
      Warm Your Engine · 34
      Interval Treadmill Run · 37
      V-PAK I · 38
      The Tour de Burn · 46
      V-PAK II · 47
      Hanging Out · 56
      Stand Up · 59
      Walk the Plank · 64
      "Rope-A-Dope" · 65
      The Home Stretch · 66
   Day Three Fitness Adventure- A Core Theme · 71
      Accelerated Interval Treadmill Run · 71
      V-PAK III · 73

The Tour de Burn- Part Deux · 82
V-PAK IV · 83
Bosu Oblique Crunches · 88
Stand Up- Part II· 90
Walk the Plank- Part II · 91
The "Rope-A Dope" Rematch · 92

Chapter Four: Transitioning to a Lifestyle of Optimal Health · · · · · · · · **93**

Chapter Five: "Know When To Fold Em" & Celebrate with Junk Food · · · · · · · · · · **97**

Chapter Six: The Next Level · **99**

Chapter Seven: "On the Road Again" · **133**
Check the "Extra Luggage" · 133
Room Service Workout· 135

Chapter Eight: Nutrition and Fitness: A One-Two Punch Against Stress · · · · · · · · · · **139**

Epilogue: Body Under Construction Tidbits · · · · · · · · · · · · · · · · · · · **141**

Appendix 1 · 143
BUC Lunch, Dinner, Dessert, and DZ Snack Recipes · · · · · · · · · · · · 143

Appendix 2 · 147
BUC Optimal Nutrition Chart (description) · · · · · · · · · · · · · · · · · · 148
BUC Optimal Nutrition Chart (weekly) · 149

Appendix 3 · 151
BUC Fitness Adventure Chart (description & example) · · · · · · · · · · · · 153
BUC Fitness Adventure Chart (weekday & weekend) · · · · · · · · · · · · · 154

Appendix 4 · 157
BUC Check the "Extra Luggage" Nutritional Chart (description) · · · · · · 157
BUC Check the "Extra Luggage" Nutritional Chart · · · · · · · · · · · · · · 158

Appendix 5 · 159
BUC Room Service Workout Chart (description & example) · · · · · · · · · 159

BUC Room Service Workout Chart · 161

Appendix 6 · 163
  BUC Nutrition and Fitness Glossary · 163

Acknowledgements · 177

About the Author · 179

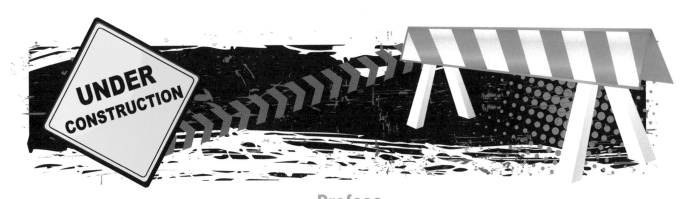

"Under Construction"

There are times, following a difficult work day, that I walk through the magnificent city of Chicago to give my mind and body the opportunity to decompress. During one particular stroll, I came across an empty lot, which had an entry blocked by two, three-foot high white-and-orange-stripped barricades to prevent pedestrians from entering the work area. Surrounding the lot was a seven-foot high metal fence on which hung a large white sign with block lettering that read "Under Construction."

As I peered through the holes in the fence, I noticed a small army of construction workers performing various tasks to clear the lot for a construction project. Excavators, with metal arm-like appendages, cleared debris while bulldozers hauled dirt away from the lot.

After several weeks had passed, I'd revisit the lot to find it cleared of debris and the construction workers using a large metal corkscrew-like object to drill holes in the ground to lay the foundation for the edifice to come.

Several months later, I'd notice a tower crane being used to lower steel beams to construction workers who used huge bolts and rivets to inter-connect the beams. Thus, the framing of the building began to emerge.

After several months, the steel beam framing was completed and machine operators are using the tower crane to assist the construction workers in setting the illustrious aluminum facade of the soon-to-be edifice. After the plumbing, electric wiring and other interior amenities are put in place, the edifice is complete. Once completed, the building is maintained by a staff of workers to assure it is functioning properly for the remainder of its life expectancy.

The edifice was not constructed over night but instead over a period of time and required patience. If, for example, I were to visit the construction site on a daily basis and observe the entire construction process, it would seem as if the construction of the building took a lifetime. However, visiting the construction site periodically made it seem as if the building was constructed in a short period.

Similarly, your body is like an edifice under construction. To lose weight, improve fitness, and attain optimal health requires time and patience as you develop better eating habits and a consistent fitness regimen. Maintaining that consistency is critical to your body functioning at its full potential for a longer period of time.

Therefore, as you build your body edifice, do not weigh yourself everyday or stare at your physique in the mirror looking for instant results. The daily monitoring will make it seem as if you are not making progress. Whether you notice it or not in the short-term, each healthy meal you consume and exercise you complete represents one more building block toward attaining optimal health.

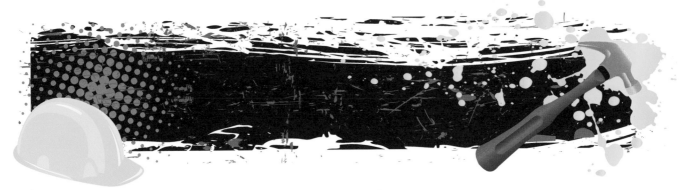

Building and Maintaining Optimal Health

Have you ever wanted to feel and look younger? Have you ever wanted to simultaneously lose weight and improve fitness, but life's daily demands have kept you from attaining these goals? Like many of you, my answer to these questions is a resounding "YES!" Yet, at 46 years old, I've built and maintained optimal health and the practical guide that I provide in *Body Under Construction* will empower you to do the same.

Many health-related books focus on nutrition or fitness in an effort to attain better health. On the other hand, *Body Under Construction* is a practical process that balances both to assist the everyman and everywoman in losing weight, improving fitness, and building optimal health. The nutrition and fitness guide described in *Body Under Construction* also can assist in reducing the risk of cancer, heart disease and other chronic illnesses that often occur because of bad nutrition and/or lack of fitness[1]. Lastly, this book discloses how nutrition and fitness can assist in reducing stress and stress-related ailments.

Body Under Construction is divided into two parts.

A nutrition regimen that includes:
- Various methods that trick your body into feeling full in order to reduce the risk of overeating.
- A nutrition plan for the frequent business traveler.
- Steps to making gradual yet significant changes to your eating habits to build and develop healthy nutrition into a lifestyle.
- How to use healthy nutrition to assist in reducing stress.

A fitness regimen that includes:

---

1 According to Toby Cosgrove, president of Cleveland Clinic, "70% of the cost of healthcare and 40% of premature deaths in the United States is from chronic disease. Most chronic disease is a result of obesity, lack of exercise and smoking…" http://www.cnn.com/2009/POLITICS/06/19/sotu.cleveland.clinic/index.html?iref=newssearch) (9/29/09)

- A three-day per week Fitness Adventure that consists of calorie-burning exercises primarily using your own body weight.
- A fitness plan for the frequent business traveler.
- Steps to develop fitness into a lifestyle.
- How to use fitness to assist in reducing stress.

Whether you are a man or woman who is 20, 30 or 40+ years of age, this book can assist you in building and maintaining optimal health.

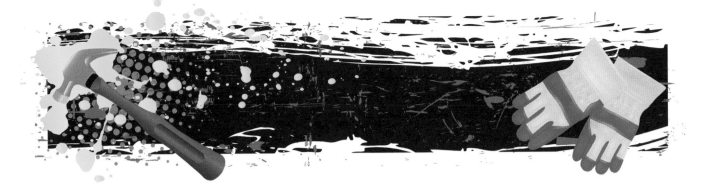

Chapter One

Getting Started

Many of my friends and family members, who are familiar with the nutrition and fitness regimen that I have maintained at 40+ years old, often ask me, "What was the most difficult aspect of developing your fitness and nutrition regimen?" Most expect me to describe a particular number of push-ups, a challenging chin-up exercise or a cold turkey-based diet plan. Ironically, it's none of these. Most stare incredulously when I state that "One of the most difficult aspects of my fitness and nutrition regimen was getting started." Getting started can be the toughest part of a nutrition and fitness regimen because it requires a change in mind and body. As a result, one of the best ways to get started is to set nutrition and fitness goals that are attainable.

Despite our good intentions, we often attempt to attain optimal health by erroneously establishing nutrition and fitness goals for ourselves that are difficult to accomplish. For example, as we enter each New Year, many of us write our resolutions and at least one is health-related. The resolution may go something like this; 'Starting January 1st I will begin to work out 7 days per week, reduce my calorie intake by 50% and lose 50 pounds in 30 days.' However, on January 1st, one revisits the health resolution and decides it's too difficult so the start date is pushed to February 1st, then to March 1st and so on until the resolution is forgotten. If the resolution is attempted, after a week (or less) the individual determines that the resolution is unattainable and eventually gives up. We become discouraged and abandon our resolution to attain optimal health before giving it a chance to work.

Therefore, when implementing a nutrition and fitness regimen, start by being realistic. Make gradual yet significant changes toward a healthier nutritious lifestyle (as described in Chapter Two and Four). Similarly with fitness, start by executing Segment 1 exercises (as described in Chapter Three and Four) and add an additional exercise over a period of time as you aim to complete a Day One, Day Two or Day Three Fitness Adventure.

As you put your body under construction by building a healthy nutrition and fitness lifestyle, it's important to remember that it took time to develop less-than-healthy eating and fitness habits and may take some time to develop new and healthier ones. So, be patient with yourself and don't give up. Additionally, do not wait until tomorrow to put your body under construction. Get started today.

Read the Label and Avoid THE 7

To attain and maintain optimal nutrition, I began to read the nutrition label on food packages. This became vitally important in not only assuring that I was consuming ingredients that assisted in attaining weight and fitness goals but avoided certain ingredients or food processes that were an impediment to those goals. When reading food labels I attempt to avoid THE 7. An easy means to re-call THE 7 is to use the following mnemonic: **F-A-T-H-A-M-R**. THE 7 includes:

 High **F**ructose Corn Syrup or HFCS: A manufactured sweetener and preservative added to various foods or beverages to preserve shelf life. Corn syrup, similar to HFCS, is a manu-factured sweetener added to foods and beverages. HFCS and corn syrup contain a high-calorie content that can contribute to weight gain[4]. They're contained in many candies, pastries, sodas and "fruit" drinks.

 Artificial Colors: Chemically produced additives used to make food appear more colorful. However, these additives may increase the risk of various health-related problems rang-ing from allergic reactions to cancer[5]. Make a conscious effort to avoid ingredients such as "Yellow 5", "Yellow 6" or "Red 40". Artificial colors are contained in certain cereals, candies, ice creams, and "fruit" drinks.

 Trans Fat: Artificial fat that is used by food manufactures to prolong shelf life. Trans fat has been known to give your body a one-two punch: It increases "bad" cholesterol (LDL) and reduces "good" cholesterol (HDL), thus increasing the risk of heart disease[6]. Trans fats are used in the production of various foods such as crackers, cookies, pastries and microwav-able buttered popcorn[7].

 Hydrogenated or Partially Hydrogenated Oils: Oils manufactured by producers to pre-serve food for longer, especially cookie and cracker products. These oils can have an adverse effect on heart health.

 Artificial Flavors: Contain a combination of chemicals to enhance the taste of food. The chemicals used to produce artificial flavors may increase the risk of various health-related

---

4 A Study from John Hopkins Bloomberg School of Public Health disclosed that reducing liquid calories especially from sugar sweetened drinks can assist in weight loss. http://www.cnn.com/2009/HEALTH/dailydose/04/06/caloric.drinks/index.html?iref=newssearch, (9/29/09)

5 Saundra Young, "Group urges ban of 3 common dyes, CNN Health, http://pagingdrgupta.blogs.cnn.com/2010/06/30/food-dyes-a-health-risk/?iref=allsearch, (6/30/2010); BBC News., "Ban artificial food colouring", BBC News/Health, http://news.bbc.co.uk/2/hi/health/3742423.stm, (5/25/2004, 3/1/2009).

6 Harvard School of Public Health, "Shining the light on trans fats", Harvard School of Public Health The Nutrition Source, http://www.hsph.harvard.edu/nutritionsource/nutrition-news/transfats/ (10/14/2008).

7 Mayo Clinic Staff (12/21/2006), " Trans Fat: Avoid this cholesterol double whammy", Mayo Clinic.com, http://www.mayoclinic.com/health/trans-fat/CL00032, (2/5/2009); University of Maryland (5/4/2007), "Trans Fats 101", University of Maryland Medical Center, http://wwwumm.edu, (10/14/2008)

problems ranging from allergic reactions to cancer. Artificial flavors are contained in certain cereals, ice creams, sodas, and "fruit" drinks.

 MSG (Monosodium Glutamate): A salt-like amino acid that is used to enhance the taste of foods. Several studies have shown that there are certain additives in MSG that cause headaches, chest pain, shortness of breathe, and nausea[8]. MSG has also been linked to obesity[9]. MSG is contained in certain Chinese food, canned vegetables, soups, and processed meats.

 Refining or Bleaching: A food process that alters the natural color of certain foods such as rice and bread. Unfortunately, the refining/bleaching process removes many of the natural nutrients in foods[10] depriving the body of the maximum nutrients it needs to operate at an optimal level. Beware of items that include the phrase bleached-enriched, such as bleached-enriched flour or bleached-enriched bread. Enriching a product occurs when a food manufacturer adds back some of the nutrients removed during the refining/bleaching process. The word enriched included on the label may seem healthy but it doesn't necessarily provide your body with optimal nutrition. Your body deserves all the nutrients naturally contained in food. Therefore, attempt to purchase food products in their most natural state For example, when selecting bread do not be fooled by phrases such as "wheat bread" that appear on the front of the package as the bread's first ingredient disclosed on the nutritional facts label on the back of the package may be bleached-enriched flour. Do not be misled by the brown color, which is sometimes made possible using artificial colors. To assure that the bread you are selecting is truly 100% whole wheat, the phrase whole wheat or whole wheat flour [11] should be the first ingredient that appears on the nutritional facts label. Consume 100% Whole Wheat bread instead of white or bleached-enriched bread because the whole wheat bread naturally includes bran and germ that provide the body with a great source of fiber. Fiber causes the body to feel full thus reducing the risk of overeating and weight gain.

Maintaining a diet that excludes members of THE 7 is just as important as exercising in the quest for optimal health.

---

8 Mayo Clinic Staff, "Monosodium Glutamate (MSG): Is it harmful?", MayoCLinic.com, www.mayoclinic.com/mono-sodium-glutamate, (1/9/2008)

9 University of North Carolina at Chapel Hill (8/14/2008). "MSG use linked to obesity". ScienceDaily, http://www.sciencedaily.com/releases/2008/08/080813164638.htm, (2/28/2009)

10 Mayo clinic staff (7/20/07), "Whole Grains: Hearty options for a healthy diet", Mayo Clinic.com, http://www.mayo-clinic.com/health/whole-grains/NU00204, (3/1/2009).

11 Wikipedia, "Whole grain", http://en.wikipedia.org/wiki/Whole_grain, (7/27/2011)

A Smooth Start

Buzzzzz! My alarm clock erupts. I attempt to locate it in the dark with eyes that are half-opened to stop the noise before it awakens my wife. It's 4 a.m. I am hungry and need to consume something that is healthy, filling and provides me with the energy to jump-start my day. To accomplish this, I consume a pre-breakfast home-made smoothie that I have prepared and allowed to chill in my refrigerator the night before. I use a blender with a 40-ounce glass jar. This provides me with enough smoothies for one 8-ounce glass each morning during a work week. With my home-made smoothie, I take an organic multivitamin to assure that I'm providing my body with most, if not all, the essential vitamins and minerals it needs to function optimally. I prefer an organic multivitamin as it does not contain artificial flavors or colors.

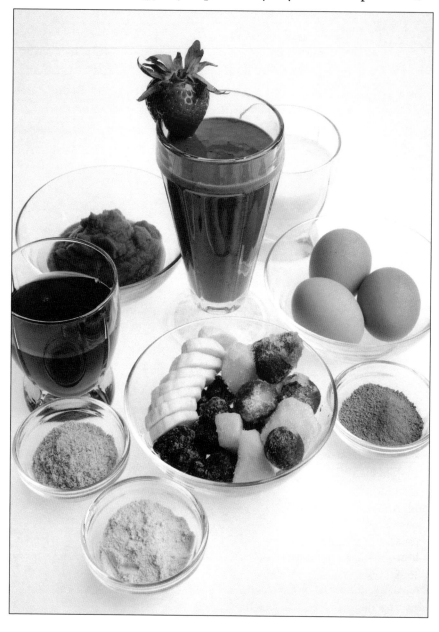

My homemade smoothie consists of the following healthy ingredients:

- 1 Egg with added Omega 3: Provides the body with protein, which plays a critical role in bone, skin and muscle tissue growth and repair[12]. Consuming eggs with added Omega 3 (which occurs as a result of the hens being fed flaxseed) provide the body

12 Star Lawrence, "Eggs: Dietary friend or foe?", Medicinenet.com., http://www.medicinenet.com/script/main/art.asp?articlekey=60421, (7/27/2011)

with more heart healthy Omega-3 than a conventional egg. When preparing your smoothie use either a white or brown de-shelled hard-boiled egg. According to the Egg Nutrition Board, "There is no difference in taste or nutrition between white and brown eggs." Getting your Omega-3 source by including one hard-boiled egg in your fruit-filled smoothie maybe more pleasing to the appetite than the Rocky Balboa approach of breaking eggs in a glass and drinking them raw.

- 1 Tablespoon berry-based powdered mix: Contains several berry extracts, including acai, raspberry, blueberry, pomegranate, blackberry and cranberry, all of which are good sources of antioxidants. Antioxidants benefit your body by fighting free radicals, which have been associated with cell damage and may contribute to various diseases such as heart disease and cancer and the acceleration of the aging process[13]. However, be sure to read the label when purchasing a berry-based powdered mix to avoid members of THE 7.

- 1 Banana: Good source of potassium. Potassium assists in the repair and growth of muscle tissue, prevents muscle cramps and may reduce the risk of high blood pressure and strokes[14]. Bananas also contain a combination of carbohydrates which provide the body with the fuel needed to function properly[15], vitamin B which serves as an energy booster[16], fiber for satiety (causing the body to feel full) and vitamin C to boost the body's immune system. Bananas also provide a thick texture causing the smoothie to become less like a drink and more like a meal.

- 2 Cups frozen berries and other fruit: One cup of frozen berries such as raspberries, blueberries, cranberries, strawberries, and blackberries, all of which are a great source of antioxidants. In addition to frozen berries, I also include one cup of other great tasting frozen fruit such as peaches, melons, and pineapples. Peaches are a good source of fiber (which makes the body feel full and reduces constipation[17]), vitamin A (for improved vision and healthy skin), vitamin C and vitamin E (an antioxidant). Melons are a good source of vitamin C and potassium. Pineapples are a good source of potassium, fiber, and vitamin C.

13 Jonathan L. Gelfand, MD, "Acai berries and acai berry juice…What are the health benefits?", WebMD, http://www.webmd.com/diet/guide/acai-berries-and-acai-berry-juice-what-are-the-health-benefits, (9/4/2010)

14 American Society of Nephrology (11/12/2008). Low potassium linked to high blood pressure. ScienceDaily, http://www.sciencedaily.com/releases/2008/11/081109074611.htm, (3/1/09); American Heart Association (9/23/1998). "High potassium diet may protect against stroke". ScienceDaily. http://www.sciencedaily.com/releases/1998/09/980923073215.htm, (3/1/2009).

15 Harvard School of Public Health, "Carbohydrates: Good carbs guide the way", HSPH.Harvard.edu, http://www.hsph.harvard.edu/nutritionsource/what-should-you-eat/carbohydrates-full-story/index.html, (9/4/2010)

16 Health Link, "Vitamin B6", © 2005-2008 Medical College of Wisconsin, http://healthlink.mcw.edu/article/985640580.html, (1/2/2008)

17 Mayo Clinic Staff, "Dietary fiber: Essential for a healthy diet", MayoClinic.com, http://www.mayoclinic.com/health/fiber/NU00033, (11/19/2009)

- 1 Tablespoon whey protein powder: A great source of amino acids which contribute to the growth, repair and maintenance of body tissues such as skin, bone, and muscle[18]. Additionally, whey protein is soluble, easy to digest and may enhance athletic performance during a workout routine[19]. However, make sure you read the label as some flavored powder proteins contain artificial flavors.

- 1 Tablespoon organic ground flaxseed meal: Provides the body with a good source of fiber, lignans and Omega-3. Fiber contributes to the body feeling full, reduces constipation, and contributes to lowering overall cholesterol. Recent studies have shown that lowering overall cholesterol may reduce the risk of late-life Alzheimer's[20]. Lignans, a chemical compound found in plants, acts as antioxidants[21]. Omega-3 provides "good" fatty acids which reduce the risk of heart disease, stroke and joint pain[22]. I prefer ground flaxseed to whole flaxseed. Whole flaxseed can be more difficult to digest, making it harder for the body to receive all of the available nutrients[23].

- 3 Cups mixed juices: Organic or all-natural juices that do not contain added sugar or members of THE 7. I include one cup of acai, pomegranate, and carrot juice. Acai is a potent antioxidant that fights cell-damaging free radicals. Pomegranate not only provides the body with antioxidants, but may also contribute to prostate and heart health[24]. Carrot juice provides the body with beta-carotene, vitamin A, and vitamin B (to boost energy and protect against cardiovascular disease[25]). Whichever juice you choose, remember to read the label.

- Half-Cup organic sweet potato puree: A great source of Beta-Carotene (a potent antioxidant), Vitamin C, and Vitamin E. The sweet potato also adds more flavor to the smoothie and (similar to the banana) provides a thick texture causing the smoothie to become less like a drink and more like a meal.

---

18 "Protein shakes: Benefits of whey and soy protein powders and shakes", WebMD, http://www.webmd.com/diet/protein-shakes, (7/27/2011)

19 Whey Protein Institute, "Benefits of whey protein", Whey Protein Institute for a Healthy Whey of Life, http://www.wheyoflife.org (9/6/2008).

20 A study by Kaiser Permanente found that "high cholesterol in midlife increased risk of late life Alzheimer's disease by 66%..." According to the Mayo Clinic, nuts, olive oil, fish, Omega 3s, fruit, fiber, whole grain and vegetables can contribute to a lower overall cholesterol level. http://xnet.kp.org/newscenter/pressreleases/nat/2009/080409cholesteroldementia.html, (10/1/09), http://www.mayoclinic.com/health/cholesterol/CL00002/NSECTIONGROUP=2, (10/1/09)

21 Wikipedia, "Lignans", Wikimedia Foundation, Inc., http://en.wikipedia.org/wiki/Lignan, (8/29/2010)

22 Colette Bouchez, "Good fat, bad fat: The facts about Omega-3", ©2005 WebMD- Women's Health, http://women.webmd.com/features/omega-3-fatty-acids, (10/28/2008)

23 Katherine Zeratsky, R.D., L.D. (1/19/2008), " Does ground flaxseed have more benefits than whole flaxseed, Mayoclinic.com, http://www.mayoclinic.com/health/flaxseed/AN01258, (5/13/2009)

24 Harvard Medical School (April 2007). "Health benefits of pomegranate juice on prostate cancer and the heart", Harvard Health Publications, https://www.health.harvard.edu/press_releases/health-benefit-of-pomegranate-juice, (3/26/09)

25 Healthy Goji Vitamin Chart-Common Health Benefits and Recommended Amounts, © 2006 Health Goji, http://www.health-goji-juice.com/vitamin-chart.html, (1/15/09)

ǁ Half-Cup Vitamin D fortified skim or 1% milk: Consuming vitamin D fortified milk reduces the risk of vitamin D deficiency which has been associated with osteoporosis, high blood pressure, heart disease, obesity, and certain cancers[26]. It also promotes strong teeth and bones[27].

Consuming a healthy homemade smoothie provides your body with a great source of vitamins and minerals, reduces morning hunger, and can give you a "smooth" start to your day.

Add Cereal to Your Fruit

One to two hours after the pre-breakfast smoothie, I consume cereal and fruit for my main course. Like many of you, I've spent most of my life filling my bowl with cereal (which typically contained members of THE 7) and adding one sliced banana on top. However, as I became more health conscience, I prepared my cereal bowl differently. Instead of adding fruit to my cereal, I add cereal to my fruit. I fill my bowl with fresh (preferably organic) raspberries, blackberries, and strawberries. I add ½ sliced banana and a ¼ cup (or one handful) of organic or all-natural dried fruit, a good source of iron that may assist in reducing feelings of fatigue. Examples of dried fruit I add are dried cranberries, wild blueberries (a potent antioxidant) and tart cherries (a source of antioxidants and anti-inflammatory elements that may assist in reducing joint and muscle pain, the risk of diabetes and heart disease).[28] After filling my bowl, I add ¼ cup (or one handful) of raw nuts such as pistachios, almonds, and/or walnuts all of which contain fiber that assist the body in feeling full and heart healthy unsaturated ("good") fats and Omega 3. A recent study has shown that nuts may reduce the risk of late life Alzheimer's[29]. I then sprinkle 1 tablespoon of organic 100% ground flaxseed meal over the fruit and nuts, and a ½ cup (or less) of an organic or all-natural bran or granola-based cereal that is low in fat, low in sugar and contains a high content of fiber. Lastly I add vitamin D fortified skim or 1% milk. When selecting your cereal and dried fruit, remember to read the label.

Since this breakfast meal contains more fruit than cereal, the body gets more natural sources of carbohydrates. These carbohydrates provide the body with a good source of energy, but refined or bleached carbohydrates, such as those made with white flour, can contribute to expanding your

---

26 Harvard School of Public Health, "Vitamin D and health", Harvard University, http://www.hsph.harvard.edu/nutritionsource/what-should-you-eat/vitamin-d/index.html, (1/15/2011)

27 New York State Department of Health, "Vitamin D and healthy bones", Helen Hayes Hospital/NYS Department of Health, http://www.health.state.ny.us/diseases/conditions/osteoporosis/vitd.htm, (2/2004)

28 University of Michigan Health System, "Clinical study reinforces heart benefits of tart cherries"(4/28/09) UMHS Newsroom; http://www2.med.umich.edu/prmc/media/newsroom/details.cfm?ID=1124, (10/22/09)

29 A study by Kaiser Permanente found that "high cholesterol in midlife increased risk of late life Alzheimer's disease by 66%..." According to the Mayo Clinic, nuts, olive oil, fish, Omega 3, fruit, fiber, whole grain and vegetables can contribute to a lower cholesterol level. http://xnet.kp.org/newscenter/pressreleases/nat/2009/080409cholesteroldementia.html, (10/1/09), http://www.mayoclinic.com/health/cholesterol/CL00002/NSECTIONGROUP=2, (10/1/09)

waistline and increasing your overall weight. They also conceal your six pack behind a curtain of fat. Yes, you too have a six pack.

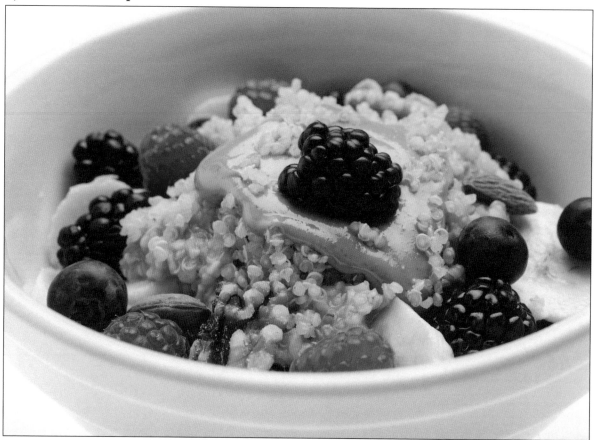

As an alternative to cereal, I add a ½ cup (or less) of cooked oatmeal. Oatmeal is high in fiber, which improves overall cholesterol, causes the body to feel full and may assist in reducing the risk of heart disease[30]. There are various choices of oatmeal available, but I prefer Steel Cut oats because it is less processed than instant or rolled oats[31] and has a slightly different texture. I also add ¼ cup of quinoa (a great source of protein) and 1-2 tablespoons of peanut butter (a low fat protein). I often sprinkle a ½ teaspoon of cinnamon which is low in calories. As with cereal, I occasionally add vitamin D fortified skim or 1% milk. Read the label of oatmeal products and avoid those brands that contain added sugar, added salt or members of THE 7.

---

30 Harvard School of Public Health, "The nutrition source- fiber…start roughing it", http://www.hsph.harvard.edu/nutritionsource/what-should-you-eat/fiber-full-story/index.html, (6/5/2009)

31 Wikipedia, "Steel-cut oats", http://en.wikipedia.org/wiki/Steel-cut_oats, (7/27/2011)

"Let's Do Lunch": The Healthy Way

Before developing healthier eating habits, my lunches were extremely high in fat and calorie content. You could probably guess what some of these meals included as they may be your favorites as well: hamburgers with all the fixings, hotdogs, french fries, etc. Although I could never get enough of these, I knew they'd hide my abs behind a curtain of fat, expand my waistline, and increase my overall weight. So, I began eating meals that were nutritious and taste great. These meals are low in calorie and fat content and are great substitutes:

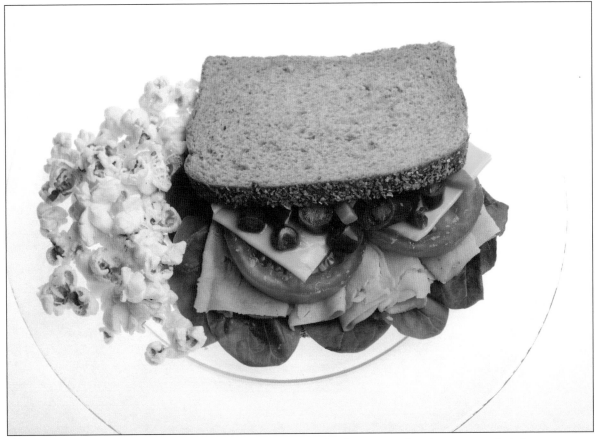

⫴ Instead of a ham sandwich with mayo, have a chicken or turkey breast sandwich:
  - Skinless Chicken or Turkey Breast: They are naturally low in fat and are a great source of protein[32] and Vitamin B. It is best to bake, roast or grill the chicken or turkey breast. Avoid frying as the Trans fat produced will offset most of the nutritional benefits.
  - Use 100% Whole Wheat Bread: Although I typically use two slices when preparing the sandwich, I occasionally will use one slice, cut it in half and use the halves to create my

32 Dr. Carrie Ruxton, "Nutritional benefits of turkey", Bernard Mathews- Turkey Nutrition, http://www.turkeyfortoday. com/features/carrie/, (9/13/2008)

sandwich. Preparing the bread in this manner limits carbohydrate intake. When the sandwich is prepared by a local restaurant that uses whole wheat rolls, I request that a third of the bread dough be removed from the inside of the roll to avoid an overabundance of carbohydrates.

- Organic or 2% milk-based cheese: A good source of calcium. Although I prefer organic cheese, 2% milk-based cheese is a good alternative as it is lower in fat content than most standard cheese. Ironically, some fat free cheeses contain several members of THE 7.

- Tomato slices: Contain lycopene, an antioxidant that fights free radicals.

- Spinach: A good source of fiber, calcium, beta-carotene, and iron[33]. My general rule is to use dark leafy greens (spinach, romaine lettuce, collard, kale, etc.) as they typically contain more beta-carotene than the lighter-colored lettuce[34].

- Organic or All-Natural Mustard: It provides the sandwich with additional flavor and is low in fat and calorie content. You also can use all-natural stone ground mustard which has a spicier taste and/or all-natural honey mustard which has a sweet taste. However, when ordering a sandwich from a restaurant, it may not offer organic or all-natural mustard. So, ask for regular mustard instead of mayonnaise which is higher in fat.

- Hot Peppers: Provide the body with Vitamin A, Vitamin C, and Vitamin K. Vitamin K strengthens bones, normalizes blood clotting, protects against osteoporosis, and contributes to restoring damaged cells[35].

---

33 Mayo Clinic Staff (3/7/2007), "Iron deficiency anemia", Mayoclinic.com, http://www.mayoclinic.com/health/iron-deficiency-anemia/DS00323/DSECTION=causes, (3/2/2009)

34 Julia Williams, "Is dark-leaf lettuce more nutritious than iceberg lettuce", Associated Content, http://www.associatedcontent.com/article/227194/is_darkleaf_lettuce_more_nutritious.html?cat=32 , (11/10/2008).

35 © 2006 Health Goji, Vitamin Chart- Common Health Benefits and Recommended Amounts, Health Goji, http://www.health-goji-juice.com/vitamin-chart.html, (1/15/09)

Instead of a standard hot dog, have a 97% fat free beef frank:

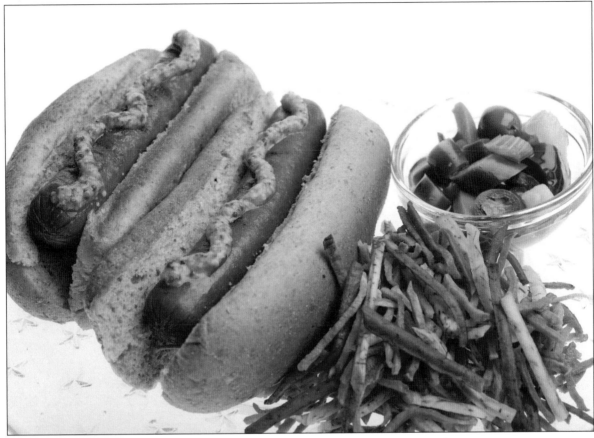

I still get a taste for a good old-fashion hot dog, but then I remember those contain approximately 180 calories and 13 grams of fat. The 97% fat free beef franks taste great and typically contain approximately 40 calories and 1.5 grams of fat. I will have one or two of these franks on 100% whole wheat bread or hot dog roll. You also can consume a "lite" "skinless" beef frankfurter. Although this frankfurter contains more calories (90) and fat content (6 grams) than the 97% one, it contains approximately half of the calorie and total fat of the typical hot dog. For condiments, I use organic or all-natural mustard, stone ground mustard, hot peppers, ketchup, and/or relish.

Instead of a hamburger, have a turkey burger (See Appendix 1 for recipe):

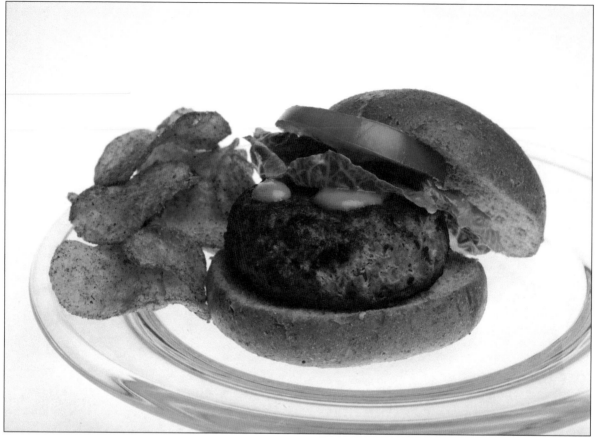

- Use 99% lean ground turkey: Provides the body with a great source of protein and contains a minimal amount of skin and dark meat, both of which are high in fat and calorie content.
- 100% Whole Wheat Bread or Hamburger Roll
- Organic or All-Natural ketchup and/or mustard: Use organic or all-natural ketchup and/or mustard (regular, stone ground, or honey) as some conventional brands contain high fructose corn syrup and hydrogenated oils. Both ketchup and mustard are significantly lower in fat and calorie content than mayonnaise.
- Romaine Lettuce
- Tomato Slices

Instead of chili with ground beef, have chili with ground turkey (See Appendix 1 for recipe):

- Use 99% lean ground turkey
- Black beans: A great source of fiber, iron, and protein. They are also a potent source of antioxidants. Although black beans contain more fiber per serving than other beans, you can use a mixture of beans (black, red kidney, lima, pinto, etc.) to prepare your chili.

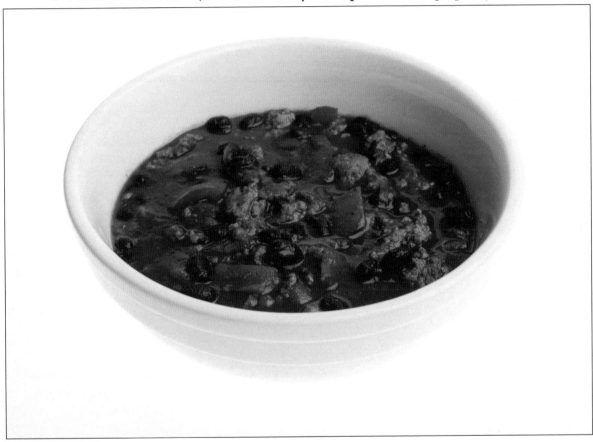

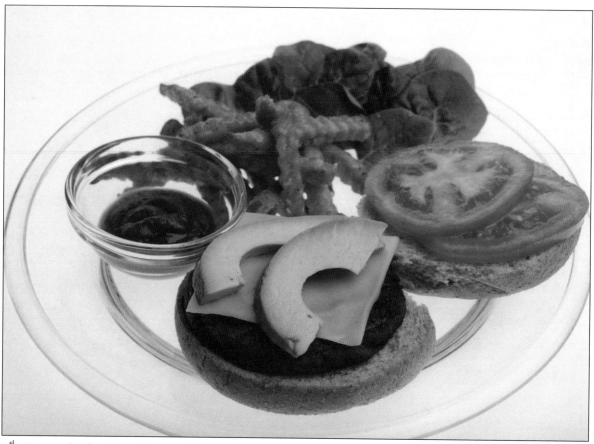

¶ Instead of a cheeseburger, have a 97% lean cheeseburger:

- A standard 4-ounce beef burger is approximately 280 calories (200 calories from fat) and 22 grams of total fat. However, a 97% lean beef burger has 130 calories (30 calories from fat) and 3 grams of total fat. An alternative to the 97% lean burger is a 95% lean burger, which contains 185 calories (60 calories from fat) and 7 grams of total fat. Both types of lean burger are a good source of iron.
- 100% Whole Wheat Bread or Hamburger Roll
- Avocado slices or guacamole: Provide added flavor and are good sources of heart healthy monounsaturated ("good") fat. When preparing my burger, I use 1-2 slices of avocado or 1-2 tablespoons of guacamole to limit the amount of calorie content consumed.
- Organic or All-Natural ketchup and/or mustard
- Organic or 2% milk-based cheese
- Tomato slices
- Spinach

If you are like me, you prefer a side snack with lunch. Instead of french fries or a bag of potato chips, choose those that are lower in fat without sacrificing taste:

‖ One handful or a ¼ cup of organic or all-natural potato chips. These healthier chips are:

- Cholesterol free;
- Cooked in peanut, safflower or sunflower oil, all of which contribute to a healthy heart;
- Contain no hydrogenated or partially hydrogenated oils;
- Contain sea salt which doesn't have additives[36].

These healthier chips come in a variety of tasty flavors such as barbeque and black pepper. But beware, they're dangerously delicious. Do not eat your lunch with an entire bag of chips within easy reach. Instead, take one handful of chips and immediately return the bag to your pantry or office drawer to avoid overindulgence. It's important to remember that organic or all-natural potato chips may be free of manufactured chemicals, but they are not calorie-free.

‖ Sweet potato fries: A good source of beta-carotene, vitamin C, and vitamin E. You can purchase raw sweet potatoes and slice them into fries. You also can purchase a bag of all-natural sweet potato fries, but make sure they are not breaded and read the label to assure that you are avoiding members of the THE 7. Oven-bake the sweet potato fries instead of frying them to maintain the maximum nutritional benefits. Consume no more than 3-ounces (or approximately 12-15 fries) to avoid overindulgence.

‖ Whole grain popcorn: A good source of fiber. You can make popcorn with relative ease in one of two ways. You can purchase a hot air corn popper. This is a relatively small and inexpensive popcorn maker that uses hot air instead of oil to make popcorn. Once the popcorn is prepared, sprinkle a teaspoon (or less) of sea salt. You also can prepare popcorn the old-fashion way by cooking your popcorn kernels on your stove using either canola or extra virgin olive oil (see Appendix 1 for recipe). Research has shown that amongst oils, canola oil has "the lowest levels of saturated ("bad") fat"[37] and canola and extra virgin olive oil are rich in monounsaturated and polyunsaturated ("good") fats. Canola and extra virgin olive oil can assist in lowering

---

36 Katherine Zeratsky, R.D., L.D. (8/27/2007), "Is sea salt better for you than table salt?", Mayoclinic.com, http://www.mayoclinic.com/health/sea-salt/AN01142, (5/5/2009)

37 WebMD, "Canola oil benefits in cooking", WebMD.com, http://www.webmd.com/food-recipes/canola-oil, 7/28/2011)

overall cholesterol thus reducing the risk of heart disease[38] and late life Alzheimer's[39]. I typically eat one cup of cooked popcorn, pour the remaining popcorn in an air tight one gallon freezer bag and store it in my pantry. If you purchase readymade popcorn, choose either air popped popcorn or popcorn products that contain no butter or cheddar.

⫼ All-natural vegetable chips: Root vegetables which are a good source of potassium and beta-carotene. I take one handful of vegetable chips to eat with my meal and immediately put the remaining bag of chips away.

The lunch meals and side dishes described above have the alluring taste of junk food without the high calorie and fat content. Consuming these healthy lunch meals are a great way to wean yourself off of fat-laden high calorie junk foods that ultimately result in weight gain.

Like many of you, I regularly had soft drinks or "fruit" drinks with lunch. Unfortunately, many of us underestimate the calories and how they contribute to weight gain. They contain several members of THE 7, such as artificial flavors, artificial colors, and high fructose corn syrup. These beverages are loaded with sugar. For example, one 20-ounce cola can contain approximately 250 calories and more than 16 teaspoons of refined sugar[40]. One "fruit" drink can contain more than 220 calories, more than 12 teaspoons of refined sugar[41] and less than 10% of fruit juice. The ingredients contained in soft drinks and "fruit" drinks can contribute to concealing your six-pack behind a curtain of fat and expanding your waistline. To lower my calorie intake, I began to read the label of beverages, changed what I drank, and reduced the size of certain beverages:

⫼ Drinking water hydrates the body and tricks it into feeling full.

⫼ A 12-ounce all-natural sparkling water with fruit juice contains 120 calories and approximately seven teaspoons of sugar (derived from fruit juice as opposed to refined sugars). Many all-natural sparkling water with fruit juice products come in great-tasting flavors such as apple, orange, blackberry, blueberry, pomegranate, and guava. Sparkling water can provide the carbonated fizzle taste that many of us enjoy.

⫼ An 8-ounce glass of 100% fruit juice contains approximately 160 calories and eight teaspoons of sugar (derived from fruit) with no added sugar.

---

38 WH Foods , " Olive oil, extra virgin", The World's Healthiest Foods/© 2001-2009 The George Mateljan Foundation; http://www.whfoods.com/genpage.php?tname=foodspice&dbid=132, (1/15/2008); Clarisse Douaud (10/10/2006), "Canola oil gets FDA heart health claim", Nutra ingredients-USA.com/Decision News Media, http://www.nutraingredients-usa.com/content/view/print/43538, (1/16/2009)

39 A study by Kaiser Permanente found that "high cholesterol in midlife increased risk of late life Alzheimer's disease by 66%…" According to the Mayo Clinic, nuts, olive oil, fish, Omega 3s, fruit, fiber, whole grain and vegetables can contribute to a lower cholesterol level. http://xnet.kp.org/newscenter/pressreleases/nat/2009/080409cholesteroldementia.html, (10/1/09), http://www.mayoclinic.com/health/cholesterol/CL00002/NSECTIONGROUP=2, (10/1/09)

40 New York City Department of Health and Mental Hygiene, "Pouring on the pounds" , press release 8/31/2009

41 IBID

⫾ An 8-ounce glass of 100 % tart cherry juice contains approximately 140 calories and eight tea-spoons of sugar (derived from fruit) with no added sugar.

Dinner: The Most Dangerous Meal of the Day

Dinner can be the most dangerous meal of the day because of the types of meals that many of us consume and the time of day that many of us eat dinner.

During my 30s, I ate meals that appeared to be healthy but actually were not. One portion of my dinner meal would be breaded chicken. I assumed that I was eating healthy because I included chicken (typically a low-fat, high- protein meat). I discovered that the breaded chicken contained more than 200 calories, 130 from fat. I would eat a side dish of instant pasta, broccoli and carrots. This combination appeared healthy, but when I read the label I discovered that it contained several members of THE 7. If that wasn't enough to impede my ability to lose or control body weight, the side dish was immersed in a cheesy or creamy sauce. The instant pasta, broccoli, carrots combination contained more than 200 calories with 30 calories from fat, more than 800 mg of sodium and 26 grams of carbo-hydrates. My dinner also included a sizable side order of white rice.

I would quench my thirst with soda or a "fruit" drink, both of which contained a prodigious amount of sugar and high fructose corn syrup. My desserts were high in calorie and fat content, and I'd have a glass of skim milk as if that neutralized it. I ate this meal late in the evening, a time of day in which I am physically inactive.

This type of dinner eaten late in the evening when the body maybe the most physically inactive, along with the natural slowing in metabolism that takes place as one ages[42], caused me to struggle with attaining weight goals. Therefore, it became increasingly important to develop healthier dinner eating habits. I developed long-lasting healthier eating habits by using the following nutrition strategy:

⫾ Ruin my dinner appetite: When I was child, my mother would cook dinner for the family. Before she finished preparing dinner she would often say, "Sloan, do not eat anything before dinner or it will ruin your appetite." Well, mom was right…again. Today I use this principle but in a slightly different fashion, ruining my dinner appetite to avoid overeating during the main course. I ruin my appetite in two ways. First, by drinking at least two 8-ounce glasses of water before dinner. This tricks my body into feeling full and reduces the risk of over eating[43]. Secondly, I eat a healthy appetizer. For example, I have a salad with vinaigrette dressing instead of the creamy dressings such as blue cheese, Ranch and Russian dressings that tend to have

---

42 John Hopkins Medicine, "Your aging metabolism…Tips on revving your metabolic motor" (1/23/2008), John Hopkins Health Alerts, http://www.johnshopkinshealthalerts.com/reports/nutrition_weight_control/1811-1.html, (6/1/2009)

43 Lori A. Greiner, "Clinical trial confirms effectiveness of simple appetite control method", Virginia Tech News, http://www.vtnews.vt.edu/articles/2010/08/082310-cals-davy.html, (8/23/2010)

higher calorie and fat content. I often include fresh berries and one handful of raw nuts in my salad. The bigger the salad the better as it will increase the probability of your body feeling full before the main course. Other healthy appetizers include broth, vegetable or black bean soups.

- Time of meal: When possible, I eat dinner immediately following a workout. The physical activity burns calories. When unable to eat dinner following a workout, have it no later than 7 p.m. to avoid eating too late. The lack of physical activity during this time results in the body burning fewer calories.

- Weaning myself off rolls: When it came to hot-buttered white rolls, I was a carboholic. I consumed an abundance of refined carbohydrates which contributed to concealing my abs behind a curtain of fat. My love for rolls made it difficult for me to go cold turkey. I put my appetite Under Construction; I set up a process by which I reduced the number of rolls I ate over a certain period of time. I started by reducing the rolls I had from three rolls to two per dinner meal during a four-week period. Once I was able to accomplish this goal, I reduced rolls from two to one per meal over the same period. As a result of the Under Construction process, my body doesn't need rolls in order for my dinner to feel complete.

- Avoid white rice: I was a carbolistic eater of white rice. I consumed an abundance of this refined-carbohydrate food. I had to first change the type of rice I ate from white (bleached) rice to wild or brown rice. White (bleached) rice is produced by a manufacturing process that removes most of the natural nutrients. Brown and wild rice, on the other hand, is a great tasting source of fiber[44]. Secondly, I reduced the rice I consumed through the Under Construction process. This included reducing my consumption of rice from a cup of cooked rice per dinner meal to ¾ of a cup during a four-week period. Once this goal was attained, I reduced my consumption to ½ a cup during the same period. I continued this process until my body became satisfied with a ¼ cup (or less) of cooked brown and/or wild rice. To compensate for the reduction, I increased my consumption of broccoli, spinach, cauliflower and/or carrots. These vegetables play a critical role in boosting the body's immune system, combating cardiovascular disease and protecting against osteoporosis. As before, gradually reducing the rice instead of going cold turkey enabled me to maintain healthier eating habits for a longer period of time and empowered me to control my weight.

- Eat slowly: I used to eat my meal so quickly I hardly enjoyed the taste. I often found myself immediately going for additional helpings, which led to overeating and ultimately weight gain. To reduce the risk of overeating, I began to eat slowly. It gives your body the appropriate time to digest the food and assist with a feeling of fullness[45]. I also take a meal halftime. Halfway through my meal I set my utensils down for 20-30 seconds. This assist in slowing the pace. After my dessert I take an after-meal break. I do not eat again for at least 20 minutes. Some studies have

---

44 The World's Healthiest Foods, "Nutrients in Brown Rice, Cooked", WHFoods, http://www.whfoods.com, (1/19/2008)
45 Kathleen Goodwin, "Successful weight loss: Top 10 tips on what works", The Diet Channel, http://www.thedietchannel.com/weightloss.htm, (9/18/2008).

shown that it takes approximately 20 minutes for your brain to comprehend that the body is full[46]. The eating technique described should be used when eating breakfast and lunch as well.

- Beware of soft and "fruit" drinks: Consume lots of water. In addition to water, you can consume all-natural sparkling water with fruit juice, or 100% fruit juice with no added sugar.
- Beware of the infamous adjectives: Stay away from packages that read breaded, fried, creamy, or cheesy. Many of these foods include trans fats, large amounts of sugar and salt and are high in fat and calories.

In addition to the nutrition strategy described above, I began to transition from high fat, high calorie dinners to lower fat, lower calorie dinners. What assisted in this transition was preparing meals that were not only healthy, but that taste great. Here are a few examples (See Appendix 1 for recipes):

- Colorful Salad: I like to make my salad as colorful as possible by including various vegetables, raw nuts and fruit. The salad includes :

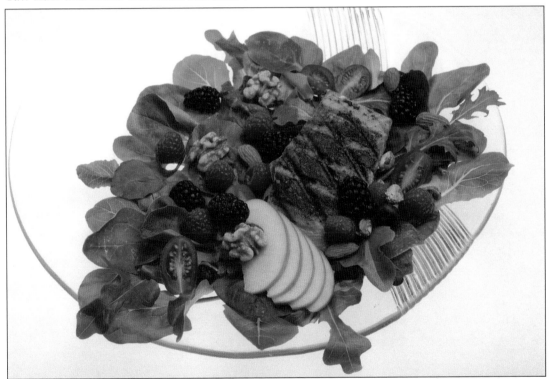

  - Spinach: Fill the base of a 25-ounce (or 750ml) bowl with spinach. As an alternative to spinach, you can use other dark, leafy vegetables such as romaine lettuce, kale, and/or collards.
  - Tomatoes: Add approximately five grape tomatoes or one sliced 4-ounce tomato.

---

46 Mark Stibich, Ph.D., "Benefits of eating slowly, About.com Longevity, http://longevity.about.com, (8/27/2007).

- Fresh and dried berries: Add a cup of fresh (preferably organic) blueberries, strawberries, raspberries, and/or blackberries. Add a ¼ cup (or one handful) of organic or all-natural dried berries.
- Sliced apples: One sliced 4-ounce apple is a good source of heart healthy fiber and Vitamin C. I remove the skin to avoid the pesticides that are often sprayed on apples. You can use organic apples, which are not treated with pesticides, insecticides, or other synthetic chemicals. You also can add oranges (blood orange, tangerine, clementine, etc.). The amount of vitamin C in oranges can assist the body in absorbing the iron contained in the spinach[47].
- Raw nuts: I sprinkle about a ¼ cup (or one handful) of raw almonds, walnuts, and/or pistachios.
- Salmon or skinless chicken breast: Add one sliced 4-7 ounce salmon or chicken breast. Salmon is a good source of Omega-3 and protein. I prefer Wild Sockeye Salmon because it contains Vitamin D[48]. A healthy alternative to salmon is skinless chicken breast which provides the body with a low fat source of protein.
- Organic or all-natural vinaigrette dressing: Add two tablespoons, available in a variety of flavors such as raspberry, strawberry and balsamic. It contains approximately 40 calories and only 2.5 grams of total fat. Avoid creamy dressings such as Ranch and Blue Cheese which typically contain 80 calories and 8 grams of total fat.

Salmon meal

- Grilled or baked salmon.
- Broccoli: A good source of vitamin C, vitamin A and other cancer fighting components[49]. I prefer to steam cook broccoli (and other vegetables) as a means of maintaining the maximum vitamins and minerals.

---

47 CDC, "Iron and iron deficiency", Centers for Disease Control and Prevention; http://www.cdc.gov/nutrition/everyone/basics/vitamins/iron.html, (2/23/2011)

48 WH Foods , " Nutrients in salmon", The World's Healthiest foods/© 2001-2009 The George Mateljan Foundation; , http://www.whfoods.com/genpage.php?tname=foodspice&dbid=104, (3/30/09)

49 Peter Jared (4/13/2000), "Broccoli beats most other veggies in health benefits, CNN.com, WebMD, http://archives.cnn.com/2000/FOOD/news/04/13/broccoli.benefits.wmd/, (7/14/2009)

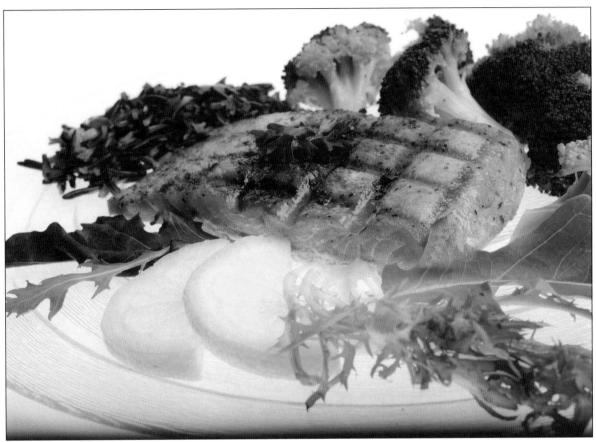

- Wild rice, a wild and brown rice combination or quinoa: Wild and brown rice are high in fiber. However, eat ¼ cup or less of cooked brown rice or wild and brown rice combination to avoid overloading on carbohydrates. You also can eat a ½ cup of cooked quinoa which is high in protein.

⫴ BBQ chicken breast meal

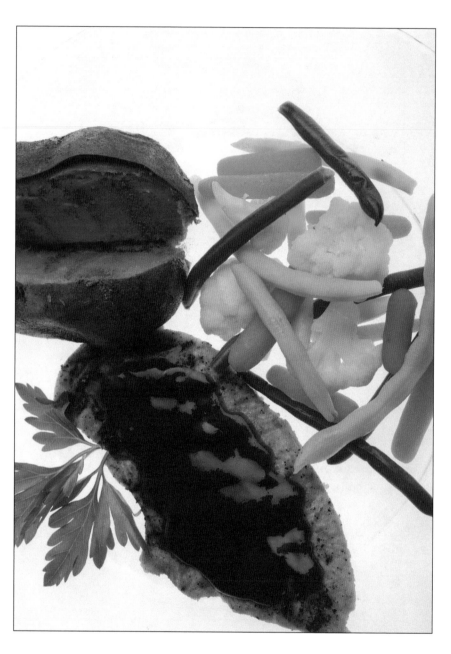

- Skinless Chicken Breast with Organic BBQ sauce: Use organic BBQ sauce which allows you to enjoy the great taste of BBQ while avoiding members of THE 7.
- Cauliflower: Good source of vitamin C, vitamin K, and other cancer fighting components[50].
- Carrots: Contain beta-carotene, vitamin A, C, and K. The antioxidants contained in carrots may reduce the risk of cardiovascular disease and cancer[51].
- Mixed green and wax beans: A good source of antioxidants, vitamin K and C.[52]
- Sweet Potato: Have one baked sweet potato. This tasty side dish contains beta-carotene, fiber, and is

50 IBID

51 WH Foods, "Carrots", The World's Healthiest Foods© 2001-2009 The George Mateljan Foundation, http://www.whfoods.com/genpage.php?tname=foodspice&dbid=2, (7/14/2009)

52 WH Foods, "Green beans", The World's Healthiest Foods © 2001-2011 The George Mateljan Foundation, http://wh-foods.org/genpage.php?tname=foodspice&dbid=134, (6/26/2011)

a good source of vitamin B, C and E. Add cinnamon, which is low in calories, for additional flavor instead of butter.

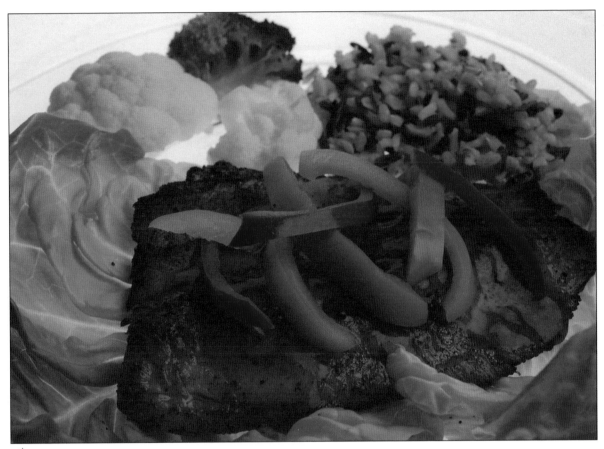

⫶⫶ Tilapia meal

- Skinless Tilapia: A source of Omega-3.
- Brown rice
- Mixed vegetables: Include a miscellany of steamed broccoli and cauliflower.

And for Dessert...

t's equally important to alter after dinner desserts as well. Keep in mind that because some of the desserts suggested are organic or all-natural does not mean that they do not contain calories. Therefore, you must monitor the quantity you consume. Eat <u>one</u> of the suggested desserts following a dinner meal. As with dinner, consume the dessert slowly.

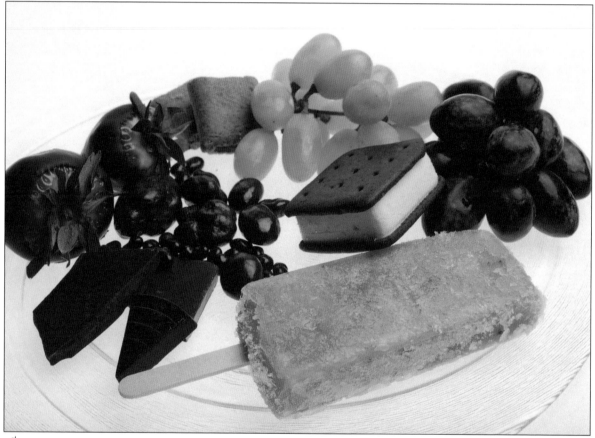

- 2 Organic fig bars: These contain 65 calories and 1.5 grams of total fat. It's a great-tasting healthy alternative to a chocolate chip cookie, some of which contain approximately 130 calories and 7 grams of total fat.
- Purple and/or green (white) grapes: A good source of antioxidants[53].
- 1 organic or all-natural ice cream sandwich: Have one 2-ounce ice cream sandwich. This "mini" sandwich contains 100 calories and 5 total grams of fat. If you are unable to find a 2-ounce ice cream sandwich, purchase a regular sized (typically 4-ounce) one and cut it in half.

---

53 WH Foods, "Grapes", The World's Healthiest Foods© 2001-2011 The George Mateljan Foundation, http://www.wh-foods.com/genpage.php?tname=foodspice&dbid=40, (6/26/2011)

⫘ 1 frozen fruit bar: This summer-like dessert typically contains 80 calories and 0 total fat grams. Purchase frozen fruit bars that contain real fruit and/or 100% fruit juice.

⫘ 1 ounce of Dark Chocolate: This dessert can satisfy the sweet tooth, appease the appetite and provide the body with a tasty source of free radical fighting antioxidants[54]. According to a study conducted by the University of Copenhagen, dark chocolate "is far more filling than milk chocolate, lessening our craving for sweet, salty and fatty food [and] gives more of a feeling of satiety than milk chocolate."[55] When possible, consume 70% dark chocolate which contains less sugar and higher antioxidant content. If you have never eaten 70% dark chocolate, you may want to start by eating 50% dark chocolate to transition from milk chocolate. Over time, transition from 50% to 65% and eventually to 70% dark chocolate. Eat one ounce or less and immediately return the remaining portion to your pantry or refrigerator to avoid overindulgence.

⫘ 2 dark chocolate-covered strawberries (See Appendix 1 for recipe): Both provide the body with a great source of antioxidants.

Danger Zone (DZ) Snacks

Danger Zones generally represent the periods between breakfast, lunch and dinner. During these periods, we can experience hunger which can cause us to become tempted to eat junk food and/or over-eat during lunch or dinner. For example, a Danger Zone during work hours is between breakfast and lunch. We become vulnerable to raiding the office vending machine which offers cookies, crackers, candy and other products that are high in calorie content and/or contain members of THE 7. Most of these unhealthy snacks provide the body with empty calories which have little or no nutritional value.

I slowly eat two or three nutritious DZ snacks between each meal. These can appease the appetite, reduce your junk food intake, and lower the risk of overeating during lunch and dinner:

⫘ Pop some popcorn (See Appendix 1 for recipe): Whole grain popcorn is a great energy source and settles the appetite. Eat one handful.

⫘ Snack on dried fruit: Not all dried fruit is healthy. Avoid dried fruit that contain artificial colors, artificial flavors and/or high fructose corn syrup. I prefer an organic or all-natural dried berry mix that includes cranberries, raspberries, wild blueberries, and sour cherries. I eat one handful.

---

54 Daniel J. Denoon (8/27/2003), "Dark chocolate is healthy chocolate", WebMD, http://www.webmd.com/diet/news/20030827/dark-chocolate-is-healthy-chocolate, (9/18/2008)

55 University of Copenhagen, "The dark chocolate version of Father Christmas is most filling", 12/12/2008; http://www.ku.dk/english/news/?content=http://www.ku.dk/english/news/dark_chokolate.htm, (11/13/2009)

‖ Fill up on fresh fruit: Grapes, apples, mandarin orange, and various berries are great-tasting alternatives.

‖ Oh nuts: I eat one handful of raw almonds, pistachios, and/or walnuts.

‖ Graze on whole grain granola: I eat one handful of all-natural whole grain granola which is available in blueberry, strawberry, cinnamon, and other flavors and is loaded with fiber.

‖ Treat yourself to trail mix: This is typically a mixture of dried raisins, cherries, berries, almonds, pistachios, and walnuts. Limit yourself to one handful and do not assume all trail mix products are healthy. Read the label.

‖ Do dark chocolate: One ounce or less is my limit. Another great tasting alternative is dark chocolate- covered nuts and dried fruit such as almonds, walnuts, berries or cherries.

‖ Chew gum: I have 1-2 sticks of sugar free gum to satisfy my sweet tooth and the motion of chewing tricks my body into feeling like its eating.

In addition to the DZ snacks, I drink at least 64 ounces of water daily[56]. It's not all in one sitting. I drink water four to six times a day using a 16-ounce container. I have two to three between breakfast and lunch and two to three between lunch and dinner. Water hydrates the body, cleanses it of waste, and tricks it into feeling full. I also drink green and/or black tea. These teas benefit the body by providing it with antioxidants and may assist in reducing the risk of stroke and bad cholesterol[57].

DZ snacks are not limited to consumption between meals. They can be eaten during other parts of the day either when you find yourself hungry or trying to reduce your risk of consuming junk food. For example, most of us experience the late-night munchies. When they strike, one or two DZ snacks such as fruit or popcorn can ease those hunger pangs. DZ snacks are also great to have when you are attending a sporting event or movie. I'll pack one to two DZ snacks in an airtight bag, such as dark chocolate, granola, and/or home-made popcorn to consume during the event. These DZ snacks are healthier than what's sold at concession stands.

Many of us consume junk food between meals not necessarily because we are hungry, but because we are bored. Before consuming food, find an activity to counter the boredom such as going for a short, brisk walk. If you continue to have a desire to eat, DZ snacks are a healthy, low fat alternative.

According to a recent study, obesity (excessive accumulation and storage of fat in the body[58]) can shorten the life span of a man or woman by two to four years while being "very obese" can reduce life span by eight to 10 years[59]. Other studies have shown that obesity among women also can increase the

---

56 Total fluid consumption can be influenced by climate, exercise, health conditions, and other factors.

57 Jeanie Lerche Davis, "Antioxidants in green and black tea", WebMD, http://www.webmd.com/food-recipes/features/antioxidants-in-green-and-black-tea, (7/28/2011)

58 ©2009 Merriam Webster, http://www.merriam-webster.com/, (3/31/09)

59 Anne Harding, "Obesity can shorten lifespan up to a decade", CNN.com, http://edition.cnn.com/2009/HEALTH/03/18/healthmag.obesity.lifespan/index.html, (3/23/09)

risk of breast cancer[60]. Improving your eating habits is an outstanding preventive medicine that can contribute to reducing your risk of chronic diseases and extending your lifespan.

Remember, however, that you are Under Construction; going through the process needed to develop better eating habits over a period of time. If during this process you completely fall off of the proverbial wagon and find yourself chowing down at some fried food joint, do not attempt to compensate by subsequently skipping meals to make up for the calories gained during your time of weakness. Skipping meals can contribute to weight gain by lowering your calorie-burning metabolism and causing you to overeat during subsequent meals.[61] Just get back on the wagon and resume your improved eating habits. Be patient with yourself and don't give up.

---

60 Roni Caryn Rabin, "Reducing your risk for breast cancer, NY Times (5/13/08), http://www.nytimes.com/2008/05/13/health/13breast.html?_r=1, (10/8/09)

61 Mayo Clinic Staff, "Insulin and weight gain: Keep the pounds off", Mayoclinic.com, http://www.mayoclinic.com/health/insulin-and-weight-gain/DA00139, (9/5/09)

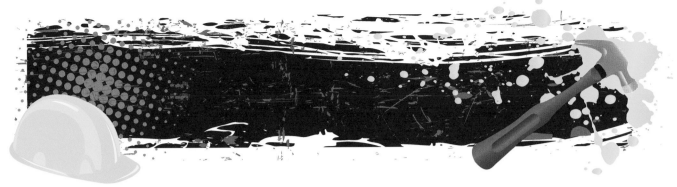

Chapter Three

Build and Maintain Optimal Health Through Optimal Fitness

A Fitness Adventure

When I was younger and single, I kept physically fit by playing pick-up basketball and participating in softball leagues. However, as I approached my 20s and 30s, my job and family responsibilities increased significantly and the time dedicated to physical fitness declined. So, I developed two series of exercises called Fitness Adventures. I call it a Fitness Adventure because of the variety of exercises. Maintaining variety will assist in burning calories, developing strength, and improving overall conditioning. It also prevents workout ennui, one becoming bored with an exercise routine. A Fitness Adventure consists mostly of exercises using your own body weight. The exercises contained can be performed at your home, a fitness center, or at a nearby park that contains monkey bars, benches and other items that can be used for exercises.

I perform two Fitness Adventures during the week and one on the weekend. I make sure my 40+ year-old body has one to two days rest in between workouts to allow my muscles recover time and reduce the risk of injury.

When selecting days of the week to workout, pick days and times that become an integral part of your regular weekly schedule. This increases the probability of performing the Fitness Adventure consistently. During the week I wake up at 4 a.m. to take a 4:34 a.m. train into the office. So, my Day One and Day Two Fitness Adventure take place after work during the week. In your case, however, your work hours may permit you to workout in the morning. Your schedule also may allow you to perform a split workout, being able to complete half in the morning before work and the other half during lunch or after work.

My Day Three Fitness Adventure, however, occurs on Saturday or Sunday mornings. Why? I spend time over the weekend to do chores from home improvement to washing our vehicles. I also invest time playing with my three children and/or assisting them with their homework assignments. So, I workout in the morning while my family is asleep. Working out in the morning gives me the physical and mental energy for the day. Working out at least once during the weekend also keeps me fitness conscious. That's critical because weekends often consist of events such as picnics and BBQs that can contribute to overeating and weight gain.

The one exception regarding the timing of my Fitness Adventure relates to the Big Eating Holidays. This would include holidays that involve large meal-related gatherings (such as Thanksgiving, Fourth of July BBQ, etc.). I often perform a Day One or Day Two Fitness Adventure the day before the holiday and a Day Two or Day Three Fitness Adventure the day after the holiday. I also take steps to assure my body is not hungry before the holiday meal. I have breakfast and lunch depending on the time of the holiday meal. I also have one to two DZ snacks and at least two eight-ounce glasses of water just before the holiday meal. By assuring that my body is not hungry, I reduce the risk of overeating during the Big Eating Holidays. Performing Fitness Adventures and planning your meals and snacks around the gatherings will keep the excess calories from gathering around your waistline.

Pre-Fitness Adventure Tips

Before providing a description of the exercises that I perform at 40+ years old, here are eight important Pre-Fitness Adventure tips:

- *Breathe regularly*: It seems obvious, but many hold their breath by clutching their lips close when attempting to complete a difficult or final rep. You may have also developed this habit and simply be unaware that you are not breathing regularly during exercise. Although there are many healthy breathing techniques that you may use, I generally prefer to inhale deeply through my nose and exhale through my mouth to provide my body with the oxygen needed for muscle recovery. I inhale during the less strenuous movement of an exercise and exhale during the more strenuous movement of an exercise. When performing push-ups, I inhale when lowering my body and exhale when raising it.

- Maintain *constant movement*: This keeps your metabolism revved up, resulting in your body burning calories throughout your Fitness Adventure. Keep seated exercises to a minimum as standing exercises typically work many parts of the body simultaneously and burn calories. Avoid long lulls between various exercises. If you are at a fitness facility and someone is occupying a workout area that you have interest in using, do not simply wait in line. Instead, maintain constant movement by doing jumping-jacks, jogging in place, shadow boxing or (if necessary) performing a different part of your Fitness Adventure. These are more efficient calorie-burning fitness alternatives than simply waiting in line.

- *Active rest*: This is the time between exercises that should last between 30-60 seconds. However, during active rest, you should maintain constant movement. You can shadow box, jog in place, perform jumping jacks or, if the mood strikes, you can even dance in place. If you are at a fitness center, you also can take a brisk walk or jog to the water fountain to rehydrate and a brisk walk or jog back. Constant movement during active rest will contribute to the body consistently burning calories. Ostensibly, shorter, active rest periods result in higher calorie-burning metabolism. However, a 30-second active rest minimum should be maintained to give the various body parts time to recover between sets. You should also use the breathing technique previously described during active rest. I use a wristwatch with a timer to monitor the active rest.

- *Constantly contract your abs*: Contract or tighten your abdominal muscles throughout your exercises and during active rest. We all have abs. They are simply hidden and this will help tear down the curtain of fat.

- *Proper form and technique*: This will reduce the risk of injury and contribute to greater strength and endurance. Five chin-ups utilizing proper form and technique can be more beneficial to your body than 10 chin-ups done improperly. Start with a lower number of repetitions if it means doing them correctly. The number of repetitions will increase over time. Review the exercise exhibits in this book every two weeks and perform your exercises in front of a mirror.

- Maintain a *moderate pace:* When performing chin-ups, for example, take one second to raise your body, pause for one second, and three seconds to lower your body. Moderately paced movements will assist you in maintaining proper form and technique in addition to building strength and endurance.

- *Don't watch the paint dry:* When I am performing time based cardio exercises on the treadmill or bike, the exercise always seems longer when I am constantly watching the timer located on the equipment. It's like watching paint dry. To prevent this, cover the time gauge with a towel, checking it periodically.

- *Consistently rehydrate*: Staying hydrated during exercise keeps the body cool, replenish fluids lost during exercise and avoids muscle dehydration, which can result in a less-than-productive workout. Drinking 64- ounces of water throughout the day keeps my body hydrated. Just before I begin my Fitness Adventure, I drink one 8-ounce smoothie and/or cup of water to assure that I am hydrated. I keep a 16-ounce water bottle within arm's reach while I exercise to rehydrate between sets. There are alternative drinks to rehydrate the body. When selecting one, be sure to read the label.

Day One and Day Two Fitness Adventure

⚹ <u>Warm Your Engine</u>

During the cold winters in the Windy City, I run my vehicle for a few minutes before driving to get the engine warmed up. This gives my vehicle's engine parts time to thaw and lubricate to function optimally. Similarly, before starting a Fitness Adventure I prefer to warm-up my body for 2-3 minutes through a combination of marching in place, light jogging in place, jumping jacks and shadow boxing. I then perform dynamic stretches. This involves stretching while moving[62] and will prepare the muscles for exercise. I perform three dynamic stretches:

- Leg swings: Using a wall or sturdy object as support, swing your leg forward (fig. 1) and backward (fig. 2) in a full range of motion 10 times per leg.

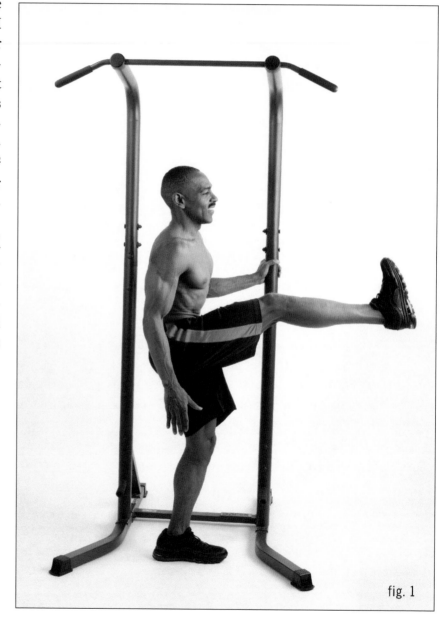

fig. 1

---

62 Gretchen Reynolds, "Stretching: The truth", The New York Times Play Magazine, http://www.nytimes.com/2008/11/02/sports/playmagazine/112pewarm.html?_r=3&oref=slogin, (10/31/2008)

- Hip rotations: Stand with your legs at shoulders width, place your hands on your hips and rotate your hips clockwise 10 times then counter clockwise 10 times.
- Arm circles: Stand with your legs within shoulders width, place your arms out from your sides and parallel to the floor. Rotate your arms in small circles clockwise 10 times then counter clockwise 10 times.

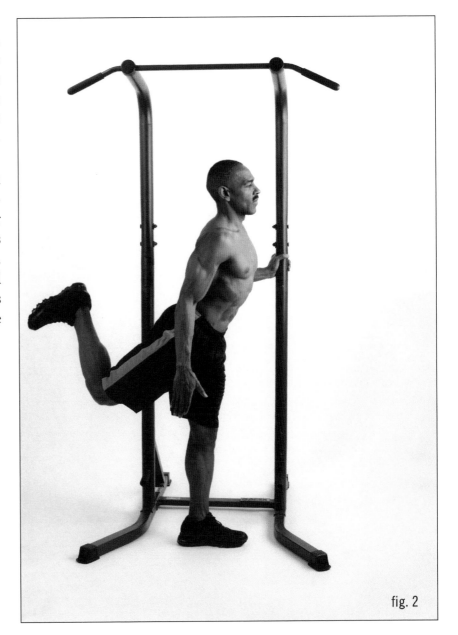

fig. 2

- Knee raises: Raise your left knee toward your right elbow (fig. 3) then your right knee toward your left elbow, while walking across the room. Do this 10 times in one direction and 10 times in the opposite direction.

I do not perform static stretches (stretching while standing still in place) as it may weaken muscles needed for various exercises to be performed during a Fitness Adventure. Instead I perform a more extensive static Home Stretch (described later in the chapter) after completing a Fitness Adventure.

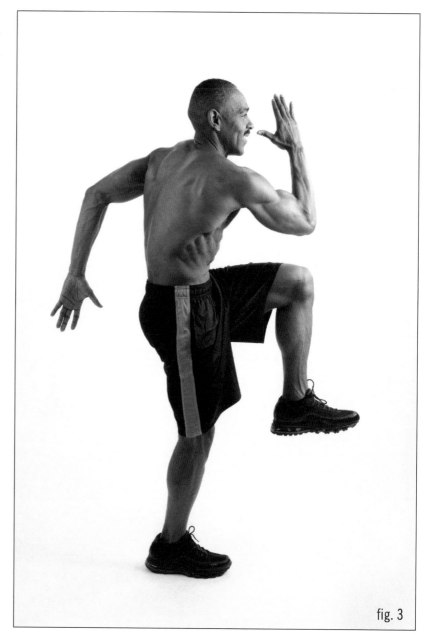

fig. 3

ᚷ __Interval Treadmill Run__

Following the dynamic stretches, I start my Fitness Adventure with an interval treadmill run. This exercise gets my heart racing and my body lubricated by working up a nice sweat. Performing the run in intervals burns calories, improves conditioning, tones the body, and reduces the risk of workout ennui.

- 15 minutes + 2: An interval run is a mixture of slow and fast-paced runs. Utilizing the manual program, I set the treadmill incline to 1.0 and the speed to a walking pace. As time progresses, I increase and decrease the speed as follows:
  - 2 minutes   speed 1.0
  - 3 minutes   speed 2.0
  - 2 minutes   speed 1.0
  - 3 minutes   speed 3.0
  - 2 minutes   speed 1.0
  - 3 minutes   speed 4.0

During the final 2 minutes of the treadmill run, increase your incline in increments of .5 while performing lowest and highest speed intervals:

  - First 30 seconds   1.5 incline   1.0 speed
  - Second 30 seconds   2.0 incline   4.0 speed
  - Third 30 seconds   2.5 incline   1.0 speed
  - Fourth 30 seconds   3.0 incline   4.0 speed

Following this exercise, I cool down by performing a 60-second slow-paced walk. Then I take a 60-second active rest.

To maintain proper form and technique, avoid leaning your upper body forward. Keep your upper body erect while running. Do not lean on the treadmill or use the arm rest for support. This will assist in gaining the full fitness benefits of the exercise. If you find that you are unable to maintain proper form and technique at the prescribed levels, adjust your speed and incline accordingly. Remember, your body is Under Construction. You're going through the process needed to attain optimal fitness, so be patient with yourself.

☀ *V-PAK I*

A *V*ariety-Pak is a series of consecutive calorie-burning exercises that work different parts of the body. When executing a *V*-PAK, one part of your body will be allowed to recover while another part is being used during the exercise. The maximum active rest between *V*-PAK exercises is 30 seconds. Remember to keep your abs contracted during each exercise and employ proper form and technique.

V-PAK I consists of a variety of pushups for toning and strengthening the upper body and bicycle crunches for toning abs. Perform *V*-PAK I as follows:

- Standard push-ups: Place the palms of your hands on the floor at shoulders width and extend your legs behind you so your body forms a straight line. Your eyes should be facing the floor and your abs should be contracted. This is the starting position (fig. 4). While contracting your abs, take 3 seconds to lower your body until your elbows are at a 90-degree angle (fig. 5). Pause for 1 second. Then take 1 second to raise your body to the start position. That is one repetition. Perform 4. Do not allow your hips to sag throughout the exercise. Contracting your glutes (muscles of the buttock) will assist in keeping your body in a straight line. Remember to inhale when lowering your body and exhale when raising your body. Take a 30-second active rest.

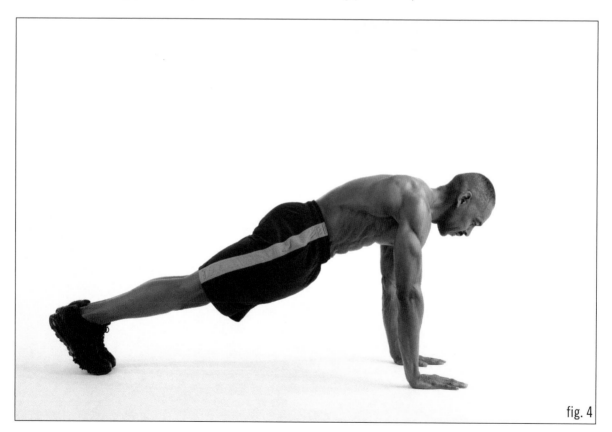

fig. 4

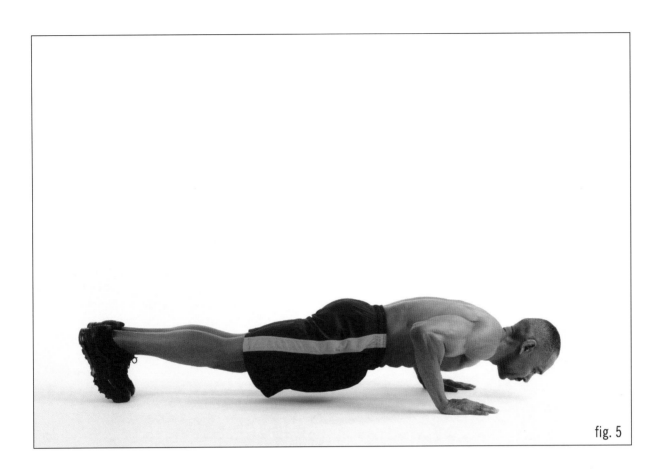

fig. 5

- Bicycle crunches: Lay on your back with the sole of your right foot on the floor and your left leg extended approximately two inches off the floor. Place your hands at the sides of your head (do not place hands behind head/neck area as this will cause you to pull yourself upward and may cause injury). Raise your head and shoulders off the floor and contract your abs. This is the starting position (fig. 6). While contracting your abs, touch your right knee with your left elbow (fig. 7) followed by touching your left knee with your right elbow. That is one rep. Perform 4. Your legs should be moving in a biking motion while your upper torso is moving in a twisting motion. Keep your abs contracted throughout the exercise. Take a 30-second active rest.

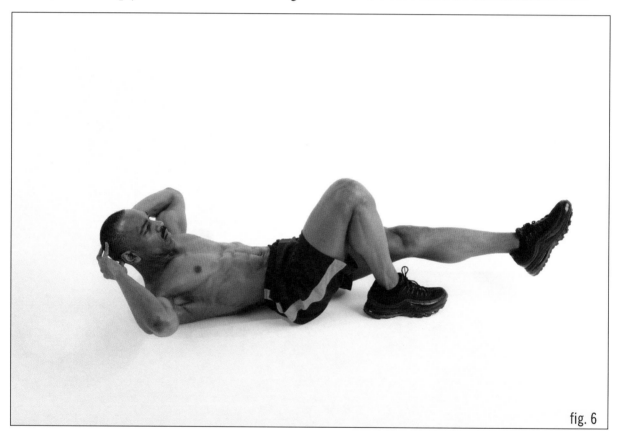

fig. 6

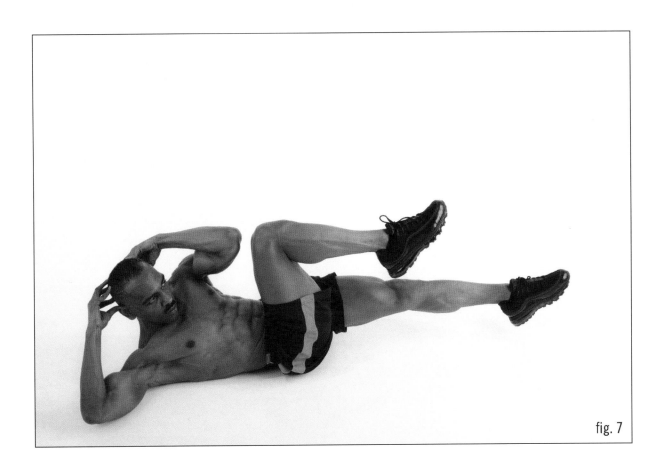

fig. 7

- Close hand push-ups: Get into a push-up position. However, place your hands within shoulders width. This is the starting position (fig. 8). While contracting your abs, take 3 seconds to lower your body until your elbows are at a 90-degree angle (fig. 9). Pause for 1 second. Then take 1 second to raise your body back to the starting position. This is one rep. Perform 3. Take a 30-second active rest.

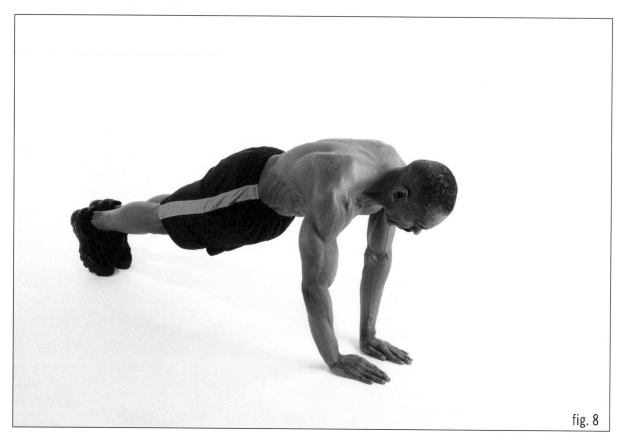

fig. 8

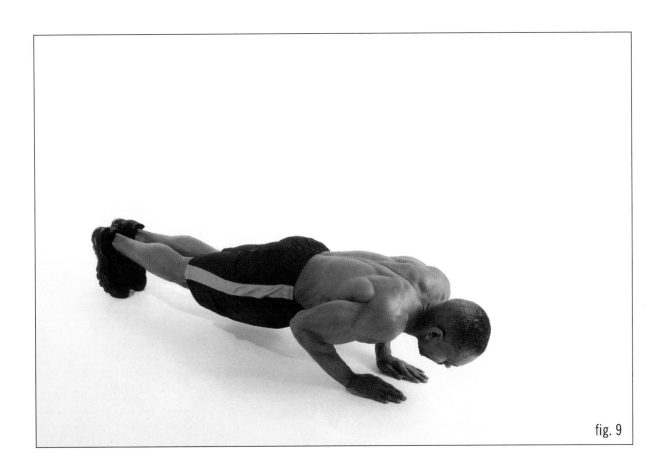

fig. 9

- Bicycle crunches: Following the active rest, perform another set of bicycle crunches. 3 reps. Take a 30-second active rest.
- Feet elevated push-ups: Utilize the same position as a standard push-up. However, place your feet on a chair or bench so your legs are elevated. This is the starting position (fig. 10). While contracting your abs, take 3 seconds to lower your body until your elbows are at a 90-degree angle (fig. 11). Pause for 1 second. Then take 1 second to raise your body to the start position. That is one rep. Perform 2. Take a 30-second active rest.

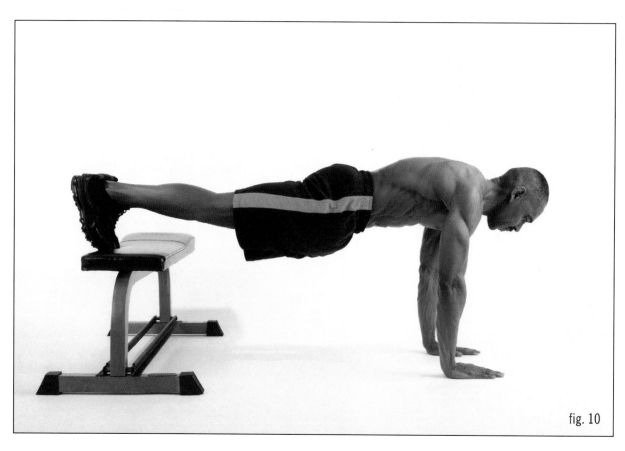

fig. 10

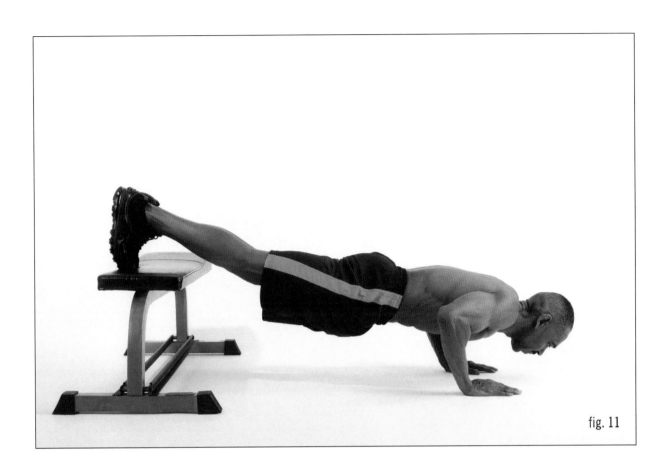

fig. 11

- Bicycle crunches- Perform another set of bicycle crunches. 2 reps. Take a 60-second active rest.

As you continue to build endurance and upper body strength, add one rep to each *V-PAK* exercise every 12 weeks.

🐪 The Tour de Burn

Have you ever viewed the Tour de France and noticed how lean yet muscular the cyclists are? Cycling is a great way to improve conditioning and burn calories and fat. The Tour de Burn is an interval bike ride.

- 15 min + 2: Similar to the interval treadmill run, the interval bike ride consists of peddling at fast and slow paces. Attach your bike to a cycling trainer. This is a relatively inexpensive devise that easily hooks to the back frame of a bike to keep it stationary. Use a cycle (or bike) computer, a small electronic device that attaches to the bike frame to monitor time, average speed, and max speed. You also can use the manual program on a stationary bike and set the time for 15 minutes. Set your bike at low gear and start peddling at a low speed. As time progresses, increase and decrease your speed as follows:
  - 2 minutes   speed 1.0
  - 3 minutes   speed 2.0
  - 2 minutes   speed 1.0
  - 3 minutes   speed 3.0
  - 2 minutes   speed 1.0
  - 3 minutes   speed 4.0

The final 2 minutes are lowest and highest speed intervals that should be performed as follows:
  - First 30 seconds   speed 1.0
  - Second 30 seconds   speed 4.0
  - Third 30 seconds   speed 1.0
  - Fourth 30 seconds   speed 4.0

Culminate the Tour de Burn with a 60-second cool down at a low speed. Take a 60-second active rest. As you build conditioning, increase your gear to medium and eventually to high and increase your speed.

The first four exercises described above are Day One and Day Two Segment 1 exercises. If you are establishing a fitness plan for the first time or attempting to re-establish (or reinvigorate) a fitness regimen, complete a Segment 1 over a 12-week period. Then add an additional exercise every 12th week until you are able to complete an entire Day One or Day Two Fitness Adventure (See BUC Fitness Adventure Chart in Appendix 3). Performing the Segment 1 exercises will not only build strength and endurance but will serve as building blocks during the Under Construction process. The interval treadmill run and bike ride will build the conditioning need to perform other upper and lower body exercises. The push-up and abs exercises will build the upper body strength needed to perform chin-up and abs exercises included in a full Fitness Adventure.

❧ *V-PAK II*

This consists of chin-ups and pull-ups for toning and strengthening the upper body and squats for toning and strengthening the lower body. Perform the *V-PAK II* as follows:

- Standard chin-ups: Using a chin-up bar, position your hands at shoulders width, palms facing your body and contract your abs. Your body should be hanging from the bar with your feet off the floor. This is the starting position (fig. 12). While contracting your abs, take 1 second to raise your body until your chin is above the bar (fig. 13). Pause for 1 second. Then take 3 seconds to lower your body to the starting position. That is one rep. Perform 4. Take a 30-second active rest.

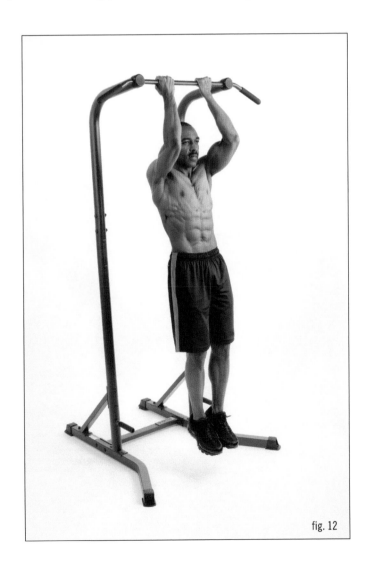

fig. 12

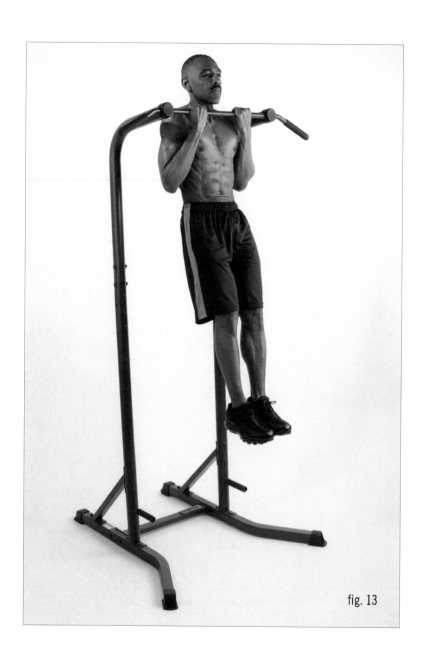

fig. 13

- 1½ Body weight squats: Place your hands on the sides of your head, position your feet at shoulders width, bend your knees slightly and contract your abs. This is the starting position (fig. 14). Keeping your back slightly arched and abs contracted, lower your body until your knees are at a 90-degree angle (fig. 15), then raise your body half way (fig. 16), then immediately return to the lower position, then raise body to the starting position (the point where your knees are slightly bent to keep tension on your thighs). That is one rep. Perform 6. Take a 30-second active rest.

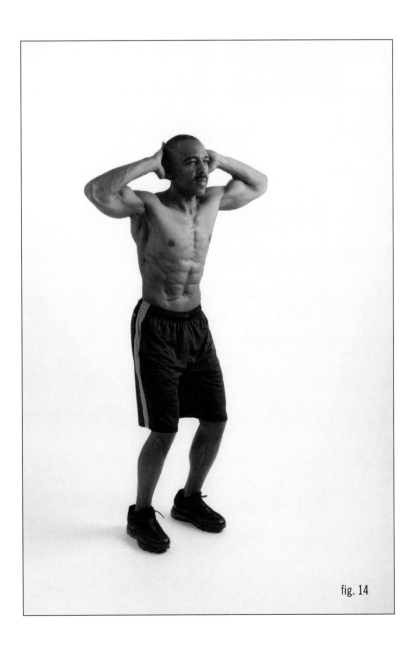

fig. 14

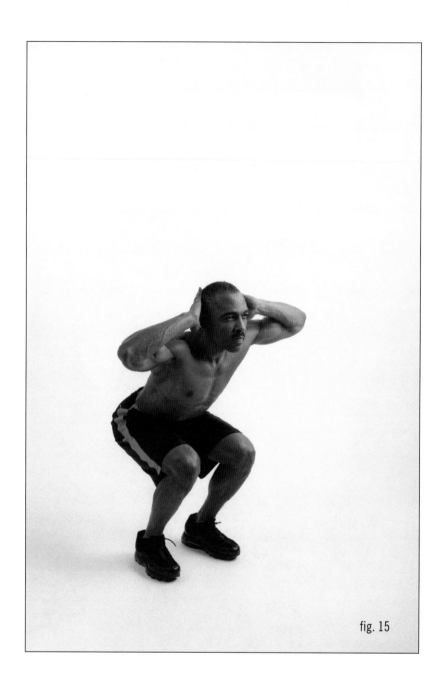

fig. 15

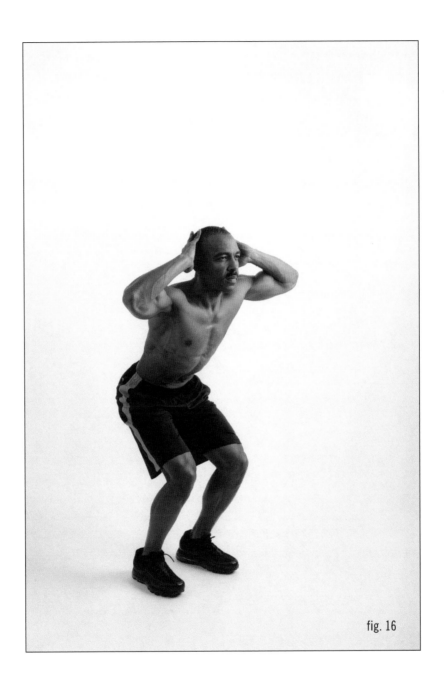

fig. 16

- Pull-ups: Return to the chin-up bar, position your hands with palms facing away from your body, hands slightly wider than shoulders width, and contract your abs. Your body should be hanging from the bar with your feet off the floor. This is the starting position (fig. 17). While contracting your abs, take 1 second to raise yourself until your chin is above the bar (fig. 18). Pause for 1 second. Then take 3 seconds to lower yourself to the starting position. That is one rep. Perform 3. Remember to exhale when raising your body and inhale when lowering your body. Take a 30-second active rest.

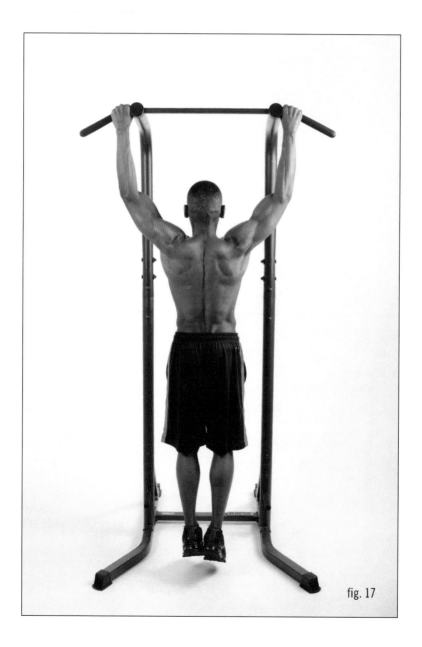

fig. 17

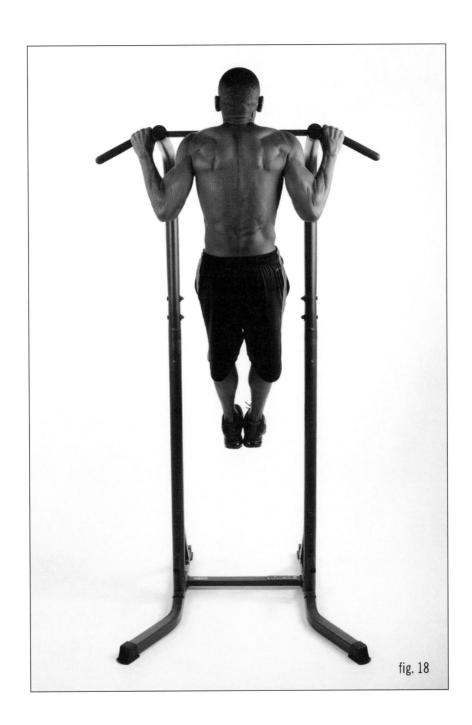

fig. 18

- 1 ½ Body weight squats: Perform another set. Do 5 reps. Take a 30-second active rest.
- Close hand chin-ups: Return to the chin-up bar. Place hands within shoulders width, palms facing your body, contract your abs. Your body should be hanging from the bar with your feet off the floor. This is the starting position (fig. 19). While contracting your abs, take 1 second to raise your body until your chin is above the bar (fig. 20). Pause for 1 second. Then take 3 seconds to lower yourself to the starting position. That is one rep. Perform 2 reps. Take a 30-second active rest.
- 1 ½ Body weight squats: Perform another set. Do 4 reps. Take a 60-second active rest.

Add one rep to each *V-PAK* exercise every 12 weeks.

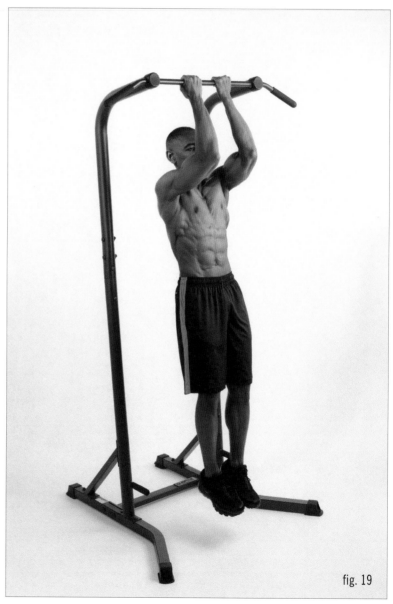

fig. 19

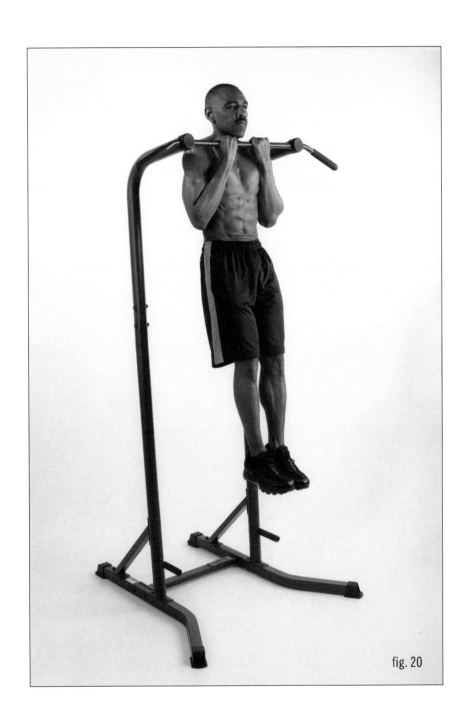

fig. 20

✎ **Hanging Out**

Maintaining variety is key to burning calories and avoiding work out ennui. After the pull/chin-up and squat variety pack, I return to a different ab exercise, hanging knee raises. Perform the exercise as follows:

- Hanging knee raises: Place each arm in an ab strap (your arms should be positioned at shoulders width) so that your body is supported by your arms and shoulders. Hold the top of the ab straps with your hands and contract your abs. Your body should be hanging from the ab straps with your feet off the floor. This is the starting position (fig. 21). While contracting your abs, take 1 second to raise your knees to your chest (fig. 22). Pause for 1 second. Then take 3 seconds to lower your knees to the starting position, then immediately begin to raise your knees again. That is one rep. Perform 4. Take a 60-second active rest. Do not allow your body to swing as you perform the exercise.

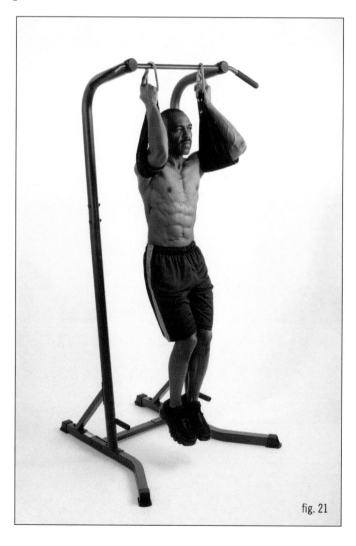

fig. 21

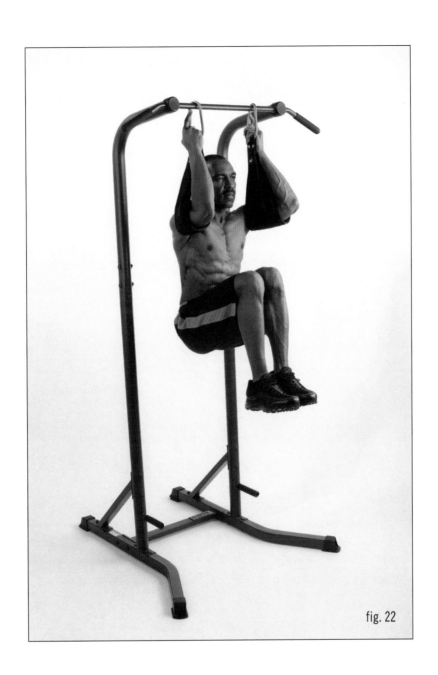

fig. 22

- Hanging knee raises with twist: Return to the starting position previously described for hanging knee raises. However, while contracting your abs, take 1 second to raise your knees to the left (fig. 23). Pause for 1 second. Take 3 seconds to lower your knees to the starting position, then immediately begin to raise your knees to the right. Pause for 1 second. Then take 3 seconds to lower your knees to the starting position. That is one rep. Perform 3. Take a 60-second active rest.

Add one rep to each variation of the ab exercise every 12 weeks.

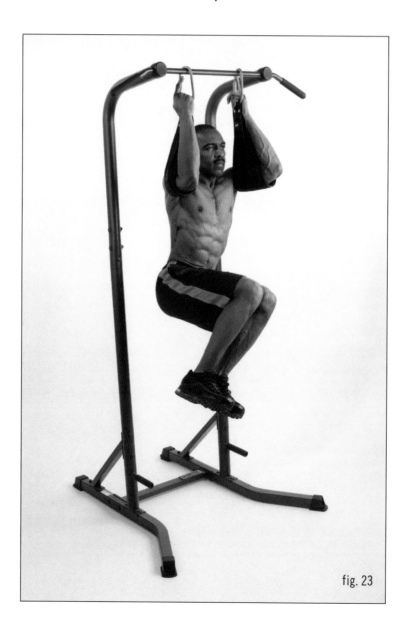

fig. 23

🔭 <u>Stand Up</u>

As you may have noticed, most of the exercises of the Day One and Day Two Fitness Adventure do not involve any weights with one exception - Curls. Curls are a great way to build and strengthen your arms which in turn provide you with incremental strength to perform other upper body exercises. Whether you are performing curls for the first time or haven't performed curls over a long period of time, start with a weight that is manageable. For some that maybe 2 pounds while for others it maybe 10 pounds or more. Starting with a manageable weight is critical to developing proper form and technique. Do not allow your arms to swing uncontrollably or your upper torso to lean back when lifting the weights as this will deny your body the full benefits of the exercise and may cause injury. Instead, keep your upper torso as stationary as possible and remember to inhale when lowering the dumbbell and exhale when raising it. To maintain constant movement and burn incremental calories, do not perform curls in a seated position. Do this exercise while standing so that the entire body is completely engaged.

- Stand-up supination curls: To lift the dumbbells from the floor, stand over them so they are positioned in between your feet. Keep your hips and chest out as you bend your knees to grab the dumbbells. Grab the dumbbells firmly and use your legs (while keeping your hips and chest out) to lift the dumbbells off the floor (fig. 24). To do the exercise, stand with your legs at shoulders width, chest out, arms close to your torso, palms facing in toward your body, abs contracted, and your head in a neutral position facing forward. Before executing a curl, raise each arm to the point in which your elbows are slightly bent so that your biceps are contracted from the start of the exercise. This is the starting position (fig. 25). Keeping your biceps and abs contracted, perform a supination curl with the dumbbell in your right hand; as you lift the dumbbell toward your shoulder, rotate your wrist (this motion strengths your forearms) so that your palm is facing upward at the end of the curl (fig. 26). Then reverse the motion as you lower the dumbbell to the starting position (the point at which the elbow is slightly bent). Immediately follow the right hand supination curl with a left hand supination curl. That is one rep. Perform 3. Upon completion of the set, return the dumbbells by reversing the steps used to lift them. Take a 60-second active rest. If you are lifting the dumbbells from a weight rack, use the same steps used to lift the dumbbells from the floor. When executing curls, take 3 seconds to raise the dumbbell and 3 seconds to lower it.

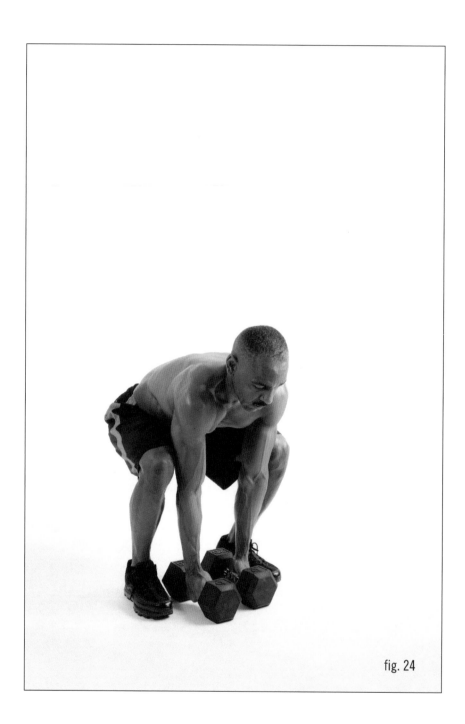

fig. 24

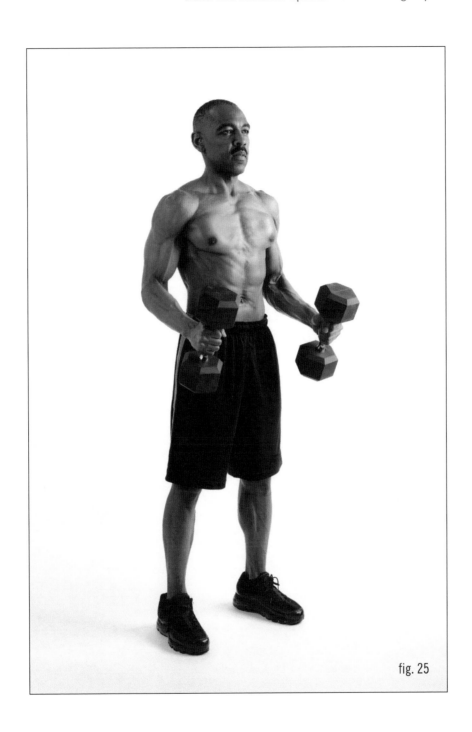

fig. 25

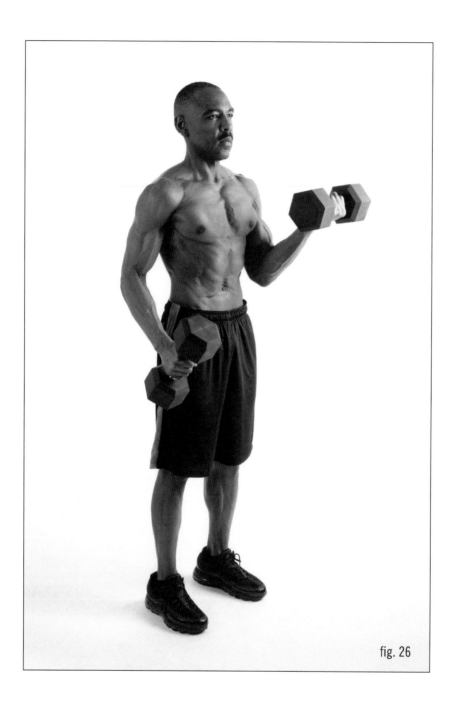

fig. 26

- Stand-up curls with palms facing in or up: To maintain variety and work additional muscles of the arms, add five pounds to each dumbbell and perform the second set of stand-up curls with palms facing in toward the body throughout the exercise for the Day One Fitness Adventure. Hold the dumbbells with palms facing in toward your body, raise each arm to the point in which your elbows are slightly bent and contract your biceps and abs. This is the starting position (See fig. 25). Perform the curl with palms facing in throughout the curl motion. Do a curl with your right arm immediately followed by a curl with your left arm. That is one rep. Perform 2. Take a 60-second active rest. For the Day Two Fitness Adventure, perform supination curls for the first set and the second set (2 reps) of stand-up curls with palms facing up throughout the curl motion. Before executing a curl, hold the dumbbells with palms facing up, raise each arm to the point in which your elbows are slightly bent and contract your biceps and abs. This is the starting position (fig. 27) Perform a curl with your right arm with palm facing up throughout the curl motion followed by a curl with your left arm. Take a 60-second active rest.

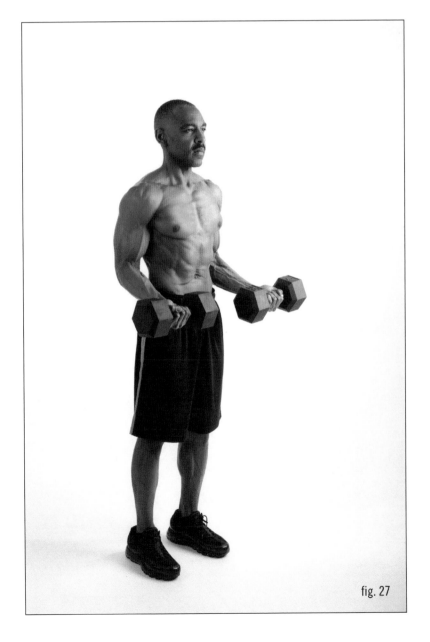

fig. 27

Add one rep to each set of curls every 12 weeks. Once you have reached a maximum number of reps (for example a first set of 10 reps and second set of 9 reps) after a series of 12-week periods, then increase the weight by 5 pounds and return to the starting number of reps. Continue this process in 12-week increments.

⚡ Walk the Plank

Although this exercise requires the least amount of movement in comparison to the other exercises described, planks can define your abs and strengthen your core.

- Planks: Get into a push-up position with your eyes facing the floor. Instead of resting on your hands, rest on your forearms with your elbows (at a 90-degree angle) positioned underneath your shoulders. Your forearms should be positioned at shoulders width (fig. 28). Hold this position, while contracting your abs, for 20 seconds. Do not allow your hips to sag during the exercise. Keep your body in a straight line. Contracting your glutes (buttock) during the exercise will assist in keeping your body in a straight line. After a 60-second active rest perform another plank. Hold position, while contracting your abs, for 10 seconds. Remember to breathe normally while performing the exercise. Take a 60-second active rest.

As you continue to build endurance and strength, add one second to each holding position every 12 weeks.

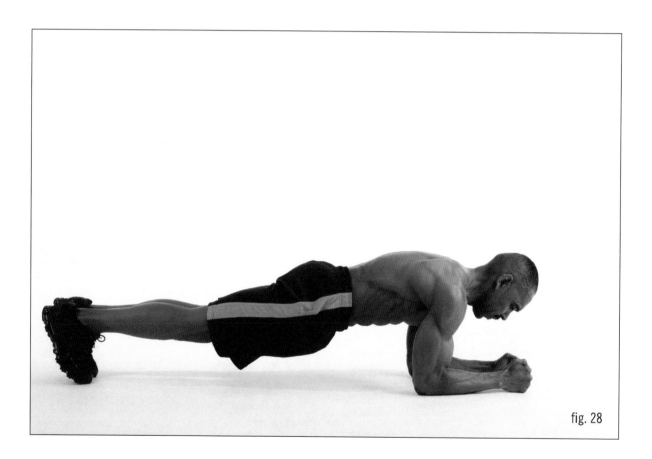

fig. 28

"Rope-A-Dope"

As a young boy, I remember my older brother and me watching Muhammad Ali train for championship fights. Although he would do various exercises to prepare for his opponent, jumping rope was an integral part of his training regimen. It played a critical role in building Ali's stamina and conditioning, allowing him to "float like a butterfly" in the later rounds. Jumping rope will allow you to burn calories and build conditioning, which in turn provides you with the stamina to do other exercises.

- Jump Rope: Complete your Fitness Adventure by jumping rope for 10 minutes. You should vary the exercise by periodically jumping from side to side and jumping while rotating the rope in a reverse motion. During the final minute, perform interval jumps - slow, then fast, then slow, then fast and so on. Cool down with a 60-second slow jump. Remember to breathe regularly and keep your abs contracted.

✎ The Home Stretch

During the Fitness Adventure, I play up-tempo music to keep my high energy level. When I complete the exercises, I start the cooling down process by playing slower-paced music during The Home Stretch. Executing a Home Stretch relaxes muscles, improves muscle growth, flexibility, range of joint motion and blood circulation.

The Home Stretch involves holding each stretch position for 20-30 seconds. You should attempt to stretch most areas of the body including:

- Legs (fig. 29,30,31)

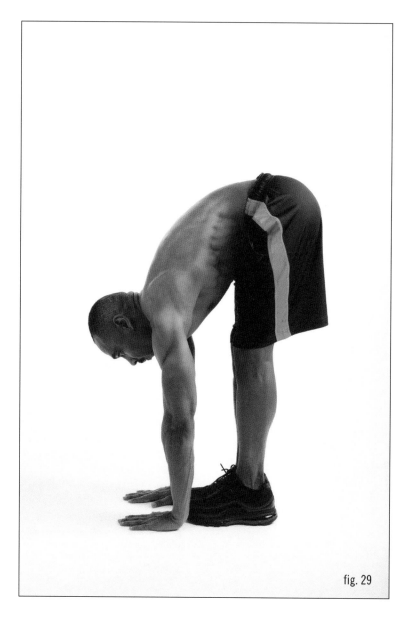

fig. 29

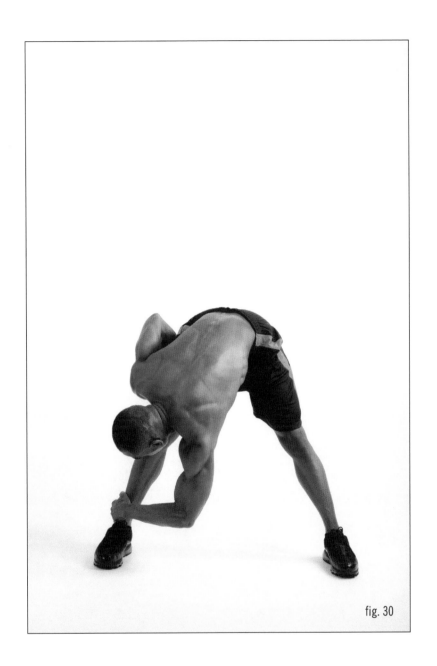

fig. 30

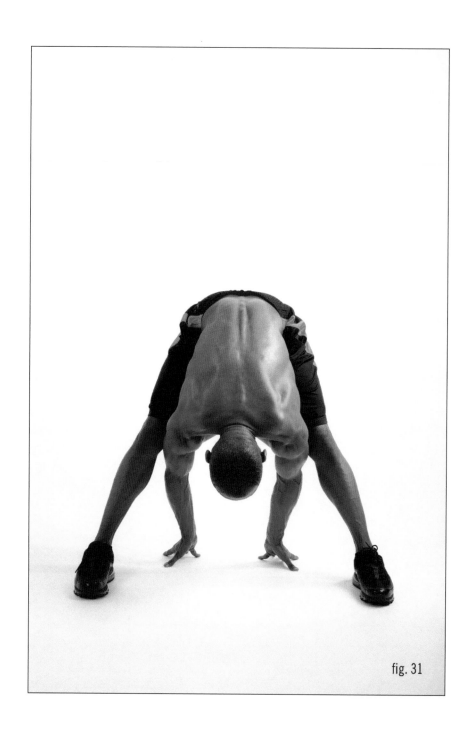

fig. 31

- Hips (fig. 32)

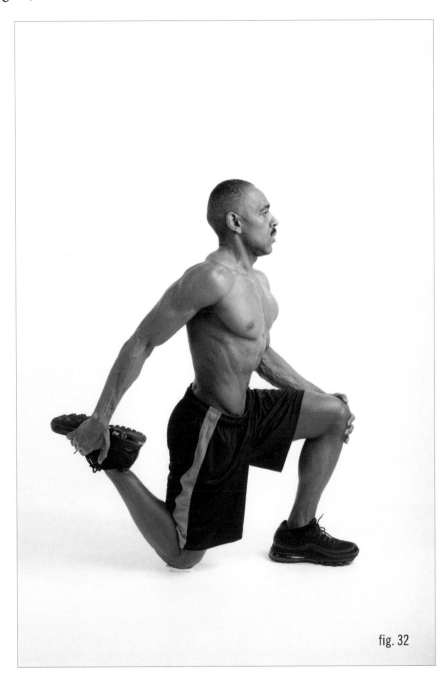

fig. 32

- Arms (fig. 33)

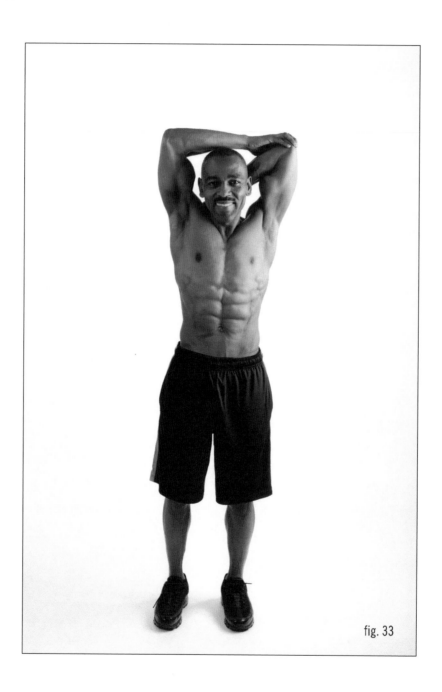

fig. 33

Complete The Home Stretch by standing on your toes and stretching your arms above your head. Hold this position for 20-30 seconds. When performing The Home Stretch, do not stretch to the point of pain or bounce when stretching as this can increase the risk of injury. Breathe deeply while holding the various stretch positions.

Immediately following The Home Stretch, take a Home Stretch Refresh, rewarding your body with an 8-ounce (or more) chocolate low fat milk. Chocolate milk is a tasty means of replenishing the body and contains calcium, Vitamin D, protein, and other nutrients that assist in the growth and repair of muscle tissue[63]. You also can replenish your body with a smoothie, water or other beverage. Whichever beverage you choose, make sure it does not contain members of THE 7. If possible, eat dinner shortly following the Fitness Adventure as the after burn can assist in burning some of the calories consumed[64].

DAY THREE FITNESS ADVENTURE- A Core Theme

My Day Three Fitness Adventure is similar to Day One and Day Two with two primary differences. Day Three takes place on Saturday or Sunday morning and includes core-stability exercises using a stability (or Swiss) and Bosu ball.

If the morning is not feasible for you simply set aside a specific time to exercise in the afternoon or early evening. You may want to implement a split workout. For example, take care of a few items from your to-do or honey-do list, then take a break from your list and perform the first half of your Fitness Adventure. Then take care of 1-2 additional items from your list, and then complete the second half of your Fitness Adventure. Unless absolutely necessary, avoid late Saturday or Sunday evening workouts as you maybe more tempted to blow these off making them more difficult to consistently maintain.

Core stability exercises involve knocking the body off balance to strengthen your core (the area that surrounds the spine, including the abs and lower back area[65]). However, since the entire body is engaged in maintaining balance, core-stability exercises strengthen other muscles of the body as well.

✎ Accelerated Interval Treadmill Run

Since I perform my Day Three Fitness Adventure in the morning, I'll consume an 8-ounce homemade smoothie as a source of energy before I start. I warm-up my body (for 2-3 minutes) as I do for Day One and Day Two then do dynamic stretches. To maintain variety for this cardiovascular exercise, the intervals are different in comparison to the Day One and Day Two treadmill run.

63 Melissa Mcnamara, (2/24/2006), "Chocolate milk...The new sports drink?", CBSNEW.com /WEBMD, http://www. cbsnews.com/stories/2006/02/24/health/webmd/main1342839.shtml, (5/13/2009)

64 Colette Bouchez (2/24/2006), "Make the most of your metabolism", WebMD, http://www.webmd.com/fitness-exercise/guide/make-most-your-metabolism, (3/1/2009)

65 Wikipedia, "Core (anatomy)", http://en.wikipedia.org/wiki/Core_%28anatomy%29, (7/27/2011)

- 15 minutes + 2: Utilizing the manual program, I set the treadmill incline to 1.0 and the speed to a walking pace. I increase the speed by an increment of .5 as follows:
  - Minute 1-2   speed 1.0
  - Minute 2-4   speed 1.5
  - Minute 4-6   speed 2.0
  - Minute 6-8   speed 2.5
  - Minute 8-10   speed 3.0
  - Minute 10-12   speed 3.5
  - Minute 12-14   speed 4.0

At the 14-minute mark, I increase the incline and speed by .5 every 30 seconds as follows:
  - First 30 seconds   1.5 incline   4.5 speed
  - Second 30 seconds   2.0 incline   5.0 speed

For the final 2 minutes, maintain the maximum incline and perform the intervals as follows:
  - First 30 seconds   2.0 incline   1.0 speed
  - Second 30 seconds   2.0 incline   5.0 speed
  - Third 30 seconds   2.0 incline   1.0 speed
  - Fourth 30 seconds   2.0 incline   5.0 speed

Following the lowest and highest-speed interval runs, cool down by performing a 60-second slow-paced walk. Take a 60-second active rest.

⚡ *V-PAK III*

Maintaining variety during your exercises works various muscles, burns calories and keeps your exercises adventurous. *V*-PAK III represents a variation on the pushup and abs exercise. It includes stability and Bosu ball push-ups and stability ball abs exercises.

- Stability ball push-ups: Get into a push up position. However, place your hands on the upper sides of the stability ball and extend your legs behind you. Your eyes should be facing the ball and abs should be contracted. This is the starting position (fig. 34). While contracting your abs, take 3 seconds to lower your body until your elbows are at a 90-degree angle (fig. 35). Pause for 1 second. Then take 1 second to raise your body to the starting position. That is one rep. Perform 4. Do not allow your hips to sag during the exercise. Your body should be in a straight line. Contracting your glutes will assist you in keeping your body in a straight line. Take a 30-second active rest.

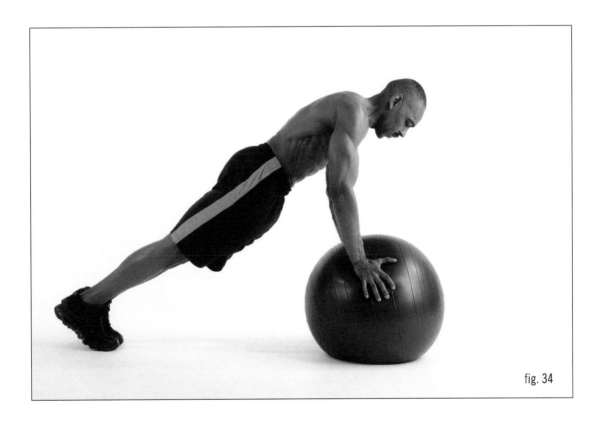

fig. 34

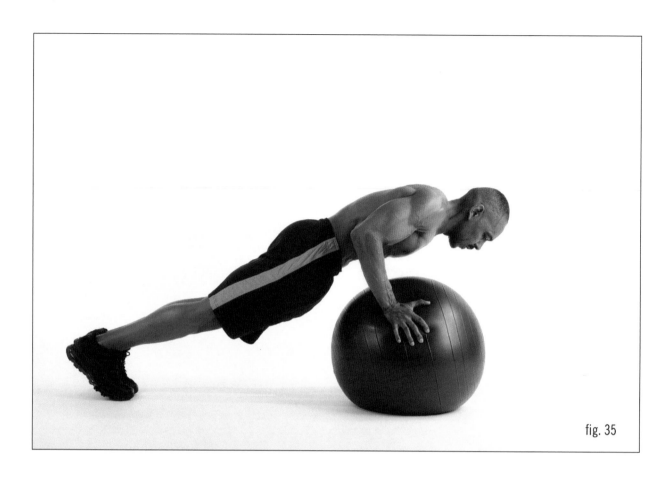

fig. 35

- Stability ball crunches: Sit on the stability ball with legs at shoulders width, knees at a 90-degree angle, and soles of your feet on the floor. Place hands on sides of head and lean back to a position that is slightly greater than a 90-degree angle to maintain tension on your abs. This is the starting position (fig. 36). While contracting your abs, take 3 seconds to lean back until your back is on the ball (fig. 37) and 3 seconds to raise your torso to the starting position. That is one rep. Perform 5. Remember to keep your abs contracted throughout the exercise and do not allow your back to bounce off the ball when returning to the starting position. Take a 30-second active rest.

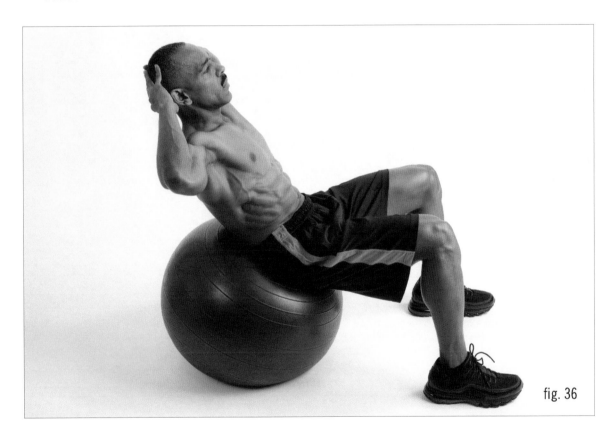

fig. 36

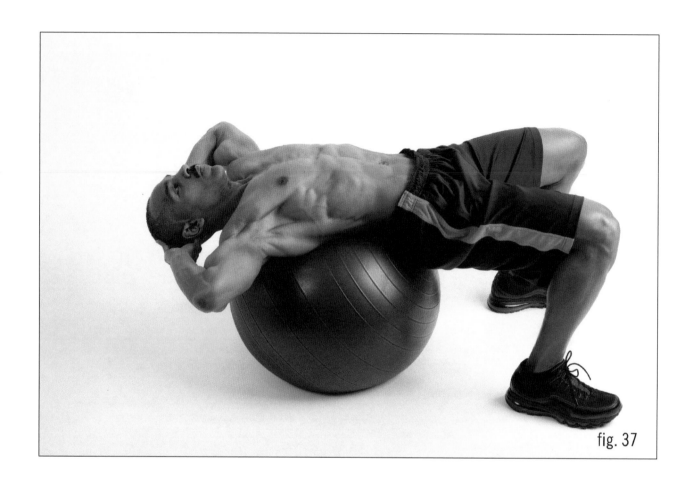

fig. 37

- Bosu ball push-ups: Position the Bosu ball so that it is lying on the domed (inflatable) side. Get into a push-up position. However, place your hands within shoulders width on the flat side of the Bosu and extend your legs behind you. Your eyes should be facing the Bosu and abs should be contracted. This is the starting position (fig. 38). While contracting your abs, take 3 seconds to lower your body until your elbows are at a 90-degree angle (fig. 39). Pause for 1 second. Then take 1 second to raise your body to the starting position. That is one rep. Perform 3. Take a 30-second active rest.

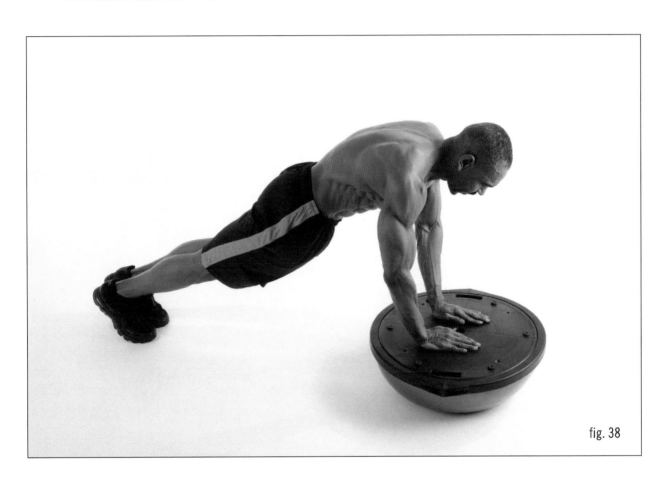

fig. 38

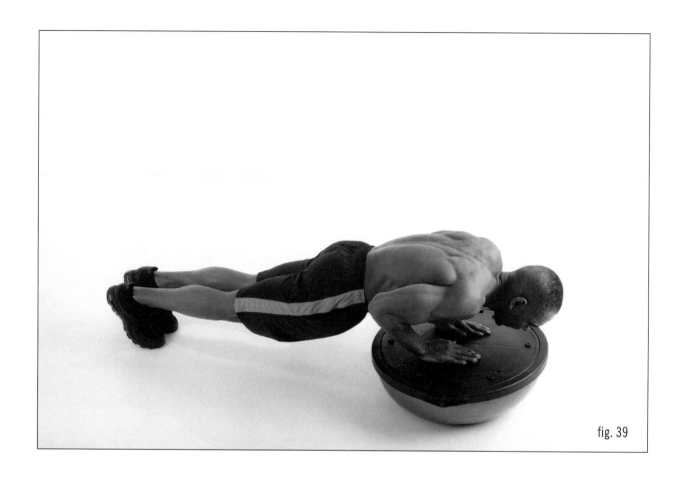

fig. 39

- Stability ball crunch with twist: Sit on the stability ball and lean back to a position that is slightly greater than a 90-degree angle. This is the starting position (See fig. 36). While contracting your abs, take 3 seconds to lean back until your back is on the ball (See fig. 37). Then take 3 seconds to raise your upper torso to the right (fig. 40). Then take 3 seconds to lean back again, then take 3 seconds to raise your upper torso to the left. That is one rep. Perform 4. Take a 30-second active rest.

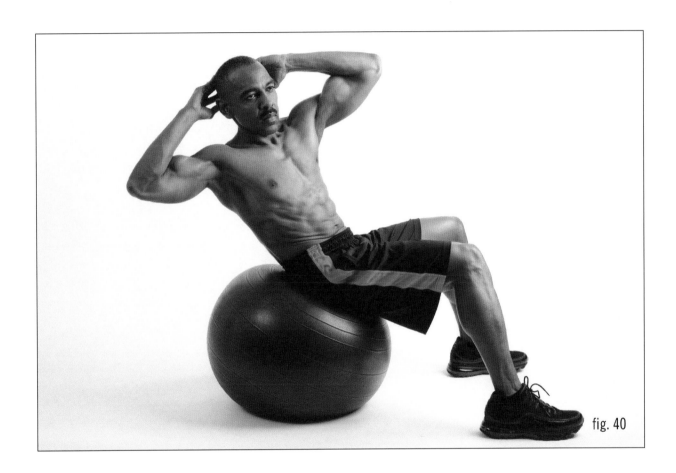

fig. 40

- Reverse stability ball push-ups: Get into a standard push-up position with your arms at shoulders width. However, position your legs on the stability ball so that your shins and tops of your feet are resting along the top of the ball, and contract your abs. This is the starting position (fig. 41). While contracting your abs, take 3 seconds to lower your body until your elbows are at a 90-degree angle (fig. 42). Pause for 1 second. Then take 1 second to raise your body to the starting position. That is one rep. Perform 2. Take a 30-second active rest.
- Stability ball crunches: Perform another set. Do 3 reps. Take a 60-second active rest.

As you continue to build endurance and upper body strength, add one rep to each V-PAK exercise every 12 weeks.

If you are performing the stability and/or Bosu ball exercises described above for the first time, lower the number of reps if necessary to maintain proper form and technique. As your core strengthens over time, you will be able to maintain balance. However, if you do not find the prescribed reps challenging enough and you are able to maintain proper form and technique increase the reps accordingly. When performing exercises on the stability or Bosu ball, wipe down the ball with a towel periodically as water and/or sweat can cause the ball to become slippery.

When selecting a stability ball size, the general rule is for those who are less than 5'0" tall, select a 45 cm-sized ball. For those between 5'0"- 5'5" tall, a ball size of 55 cm should be used. If you are between 5'6" and 6'0" tall, a ball size of 65 cm should suffice. For those over 6'0" tall, a 75 cm sized ball should be chosen.

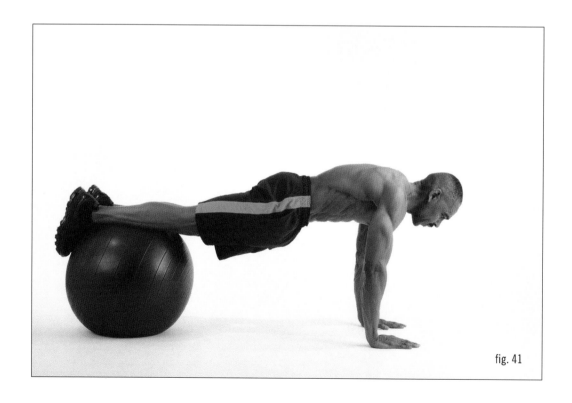

fig. 41

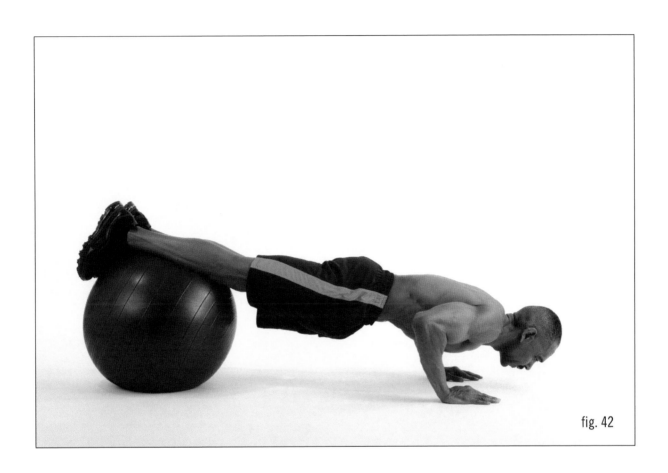

fig. 42

🏃 The Tour de Burn- Part Deux

As described earlier, the Tour de Burn is great for improving conditioning and burning calories and fat. However these intervals are sequenced differently to maintain variety for this cardiovascular exercise.

- 15 Min + 2: You can either attach your bike to a cycle trainer or use the manual program on a stationary bike. Set your bike at low gear and start peddling at a low speed. As time progresses, increase your speed as follows:
  - Minute 1-2   speed 1.0
  - Minute 2-4   speed 2.0
  - Minute 4-6   speed 3.0
  - Minute 6-8   speed 4.0
  - Minute 8-10   speed 5.0
  - Minute 10-12 speed 6.0
  - Minute 12-14 speed 7.0

At the 14-minute mark, increase the speed by 1.0 every 30 seconds as follows:

  - First 30 seconds   speed 8.0
  - Second 30 seconds   speed 9.0

The final 2 minutes are lowest and highest speed intervals that should be performed as follows:

  - First 30 seconds   speed 1.0
  - Second 30 seconds   speed 9.0
  - Third 30 seconds   speed 1.0
  - Fourth 30 seconds   speed 9.0

Culminate the exercise by performing a 60-second cool down at a low bike speed followed by a 60-second active rest. As you build conditioning over time, set your gear to medium and eventually to high and increase your speed accordingly.

The first four exercises described are Day Three Segment 1 exercises. Start by completing a Segment 1 over a 12- week period. Then add the next exercise in sequence every 12th week until you are able to complete an entire Day Three Fitness Adventure (See BUC Fitness Adventure Chart in Appendix 3).

❧ *V-PAK IV*

V-PAK IV consists of pull and chin-up exercises and Bosu squats.

- Pull-ups: Do a set of pull-ups as described earlier (See fig. 17, 18). Perform 4 reps. Remember to exhale when raising your body and inhale when lowering your body. Take a 30-second active rest.

- 1 ½ Bosu body weight squats: Stand on the domed side of the Bosu with feet within shoulders width. Place your hands at the sides of your head and slightly bend your knees. This is the starting position (fig. 43). Keeping your back slightly arched and abs contracted, lower your body until your knees are at a 90-degree angle (fig. 44), then raise your body half way (fig. 45), then immediately return to the lower position, then raise your body to the starting position. That is one rep. Perform 6. Take a 30-second active rest. When performing exercises on the Bosu, wipe down the ball periodically with a towel as water and/or sweat can cause the ball to become slippery. You may drape a towel over the domed side of the Bosu to keep the ball dry during the exercise.

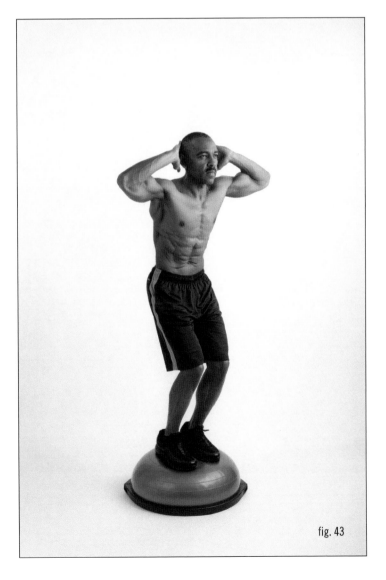

fig. 43

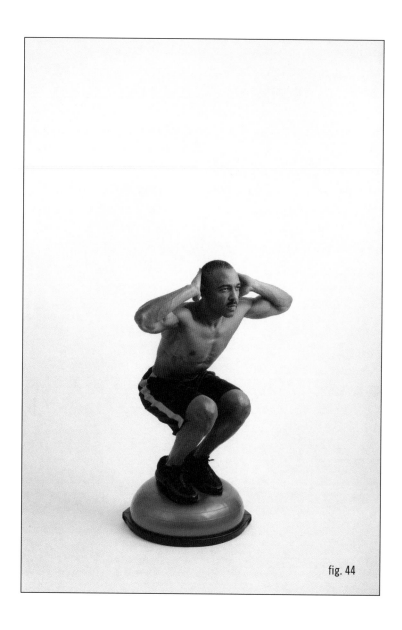

fig. 44

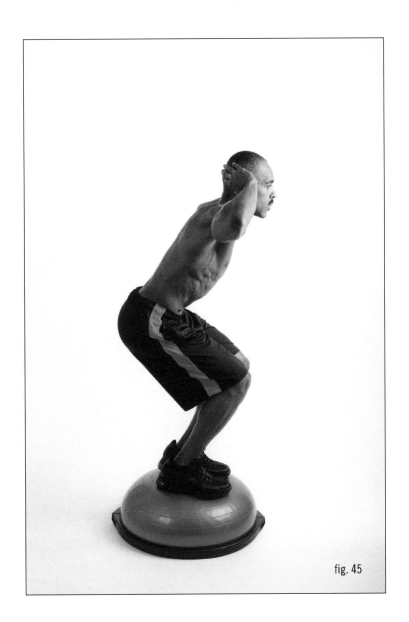

fig. 45

- Standard chin-ups: Do a set of standard chin-ups as described earlier (See fig. 12, 13). Perform 3 reps. Take a 30-second active rest.
- 1 ½ Bosu body weight squats: Do another set; 5 reps. Take a 30-second active rest.
- Close hand pull-ups: Return to the chin-up bar. Position your hands within shoulders width, palms facing away from your body and contract your abs. Your body should be hanging from the bar with your feet off the floor. This is the starting position (fig. 46). While contracting your abs, take 1 second to raise your body until your chin is above the bar (fig. 47). Pause for 1 second. Then take 3 seconds to lower your body to the starting position. That is one rep. Perform 2. Take a 30-second active rest.
- 1 ½ Bosu body weight squats: Do another set; 4 reps. Take a 60-second active rest.

Add one rep to each *V*-PAK exercise every 12 weeks.

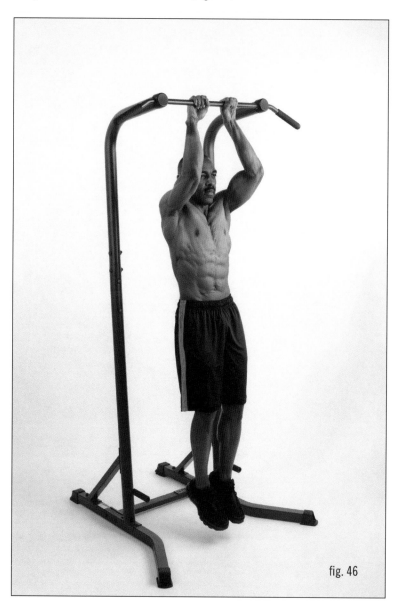

fig. 46

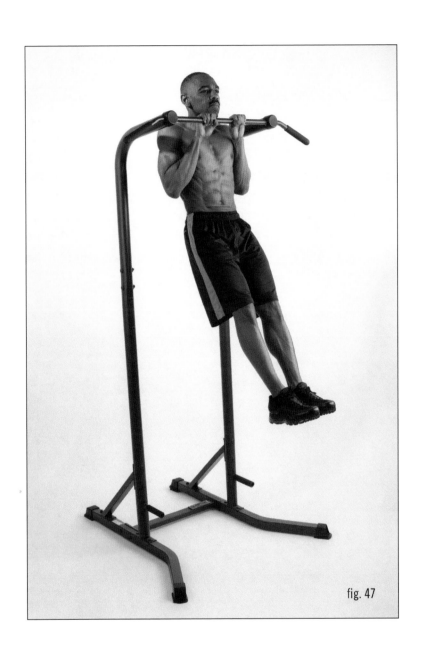

fig. 47

🏃 **<u>Bosu Oblique Crunches</u>**

This variation on the crunch will assist in defining your oblique muscles- located along your torso- while simultaneously developing your core.

- Bosu oblique crunches: Using a Bosu ball, lay on your left side with your hip approximately one inch from the top of the inflatable side of the Bosu. With your hip leaning into the Bosu, cross your ankles, place your hands on the sides of your head, keep your elbows out, and contract your abs. This is the starting position (fig. 48). While contracting your abs, raise your upper torso until your oblique muscles are fully contracted (fig. 49) then lower your upper torso to the starting position. That is one rep. Perform 5. Immediately perform the same exercise lying on the right side of your body. Perform 5. After a 60-second active rest, perform 4 reps lying on your left side immediately followed by 4 reps lying on your right side. Take a 60 second active rest.

Add one rep to each set every 12 weeks.

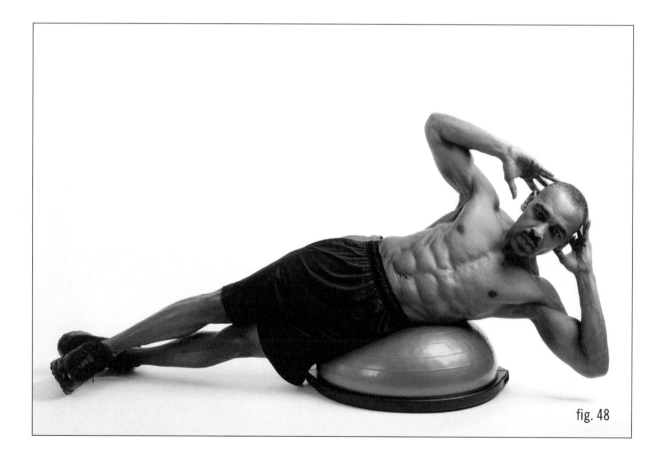

fig. 48

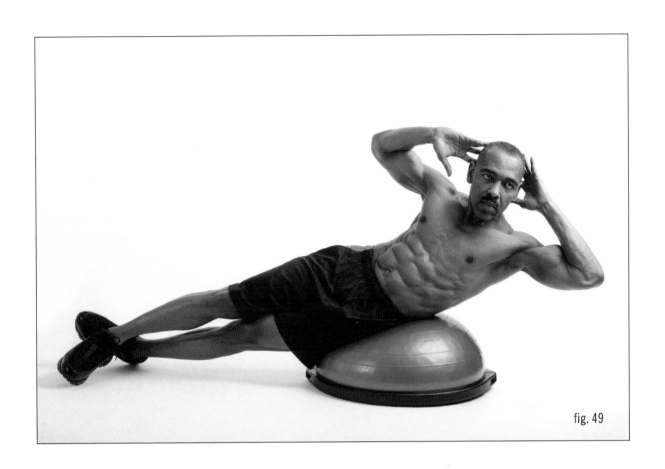

fig. 49

Stand Up - Part II

- Stand up curls with palms facing in: Do a set of stand-up curls with palms facing in toward the body throughout the curl motion as described earlier (See fig. 25 for starting position). Perform 3 reps. Take a 60-second active rest.

- Stand up curls with palms facing up: Perform another set of curls at a heavier weight (add 5 pounds to each dumbbell). Hold dumbbells with palms facing up throughout the curl motion as described earlier (See fig. 27 for starting position). Perform 2 reps. Take a 60-second active rest. When executing curls, take 3 seconds to raise the dumbbell and 3 seconds to lower it.

Add one rep to each set of curls every 12 weeks. Once you have reached a maximum number of reps (for example a first set of 10 reps and second set of 9 reps) following a series of 12-week periods, then increase the weight by 5 pounds and return to the starting number of reps (for example, first set of 3 reps and second set of 2 reps). Continue this process in increments of 12 weeks.

🔾 Walk the Plank- Part II

This is a plank exercise with the use of a stability ball. This exercise will not only assist in defining your abs and strengthening your core but will develop your legs, shoulders and other muscles that are used to maintain balance on the ball.

- Stability ball planks: Get into a normal plank position, but instead of resting your forearms on the floor, rest your forearms on the top of the stability ball. Contract your abs and keep your body in a straight line (fig. 50). Hold the position for 20 seconds. Contracting your glutes (buttock) will assist in keeping your body in a straight line. Do not allow your hips to sag during the exercise and breathe normally. After a 60-second active rest, perform another set by holding the position for 10 seconds. Take a 60-second active rest.

Add one second to each set of planks every 12 weeks.

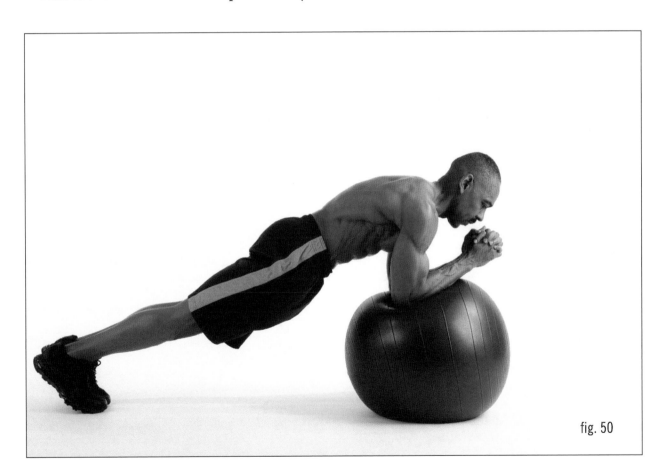

fig. 50

The "Rope-A-Dope" Rematch

Jump Rope: Complete your Fitness Adventure by jumping rope for 10 minutes. You should vary the exercise by periodically jumping from side to side and jumping while rotating the rope in reverse motion. During the final minute, perform interval jumps- slow, then fast, then slow, then fast and so on. Cool down with a 60-second slow jump. Remember to breathe regularly and keep your abs contracted during the exercise. After this exercise perform The Home Stretch and take a Home Stretch Refresh: replenish your body with an 8-ounce (or more) chocolate low fat milk, smoothie or other beverage.

Implementing a consistent fitness regimen whether you are 20, 30 or 40+ is an outstanding form of preventive medicine against chronic illnesses[66] such as cancer (including breast cancer among women[67]) and heart disease (the leading cause of death for men[68] and women[69] in the United States). However, as you develop your consistent fitness regimen, remember that you are Under Construction. If during this process you fall off the proverbial wagon by skipping a Day One, Day Two or Day Three Fitness Adventure, do not punish yourself, for example, by working out two consecutive days to make up for the workout missed. This may cause injury and discourage you from re-establishing your fitness regimen. Instead, simply resume with a Day One, Day Two or Day Three Fitness Adventure. Be patient with yourself and don't give up.

---

66 According to Toby Cosgrove, president of Cleveland Clinic "70% of the cost in healthcare is from chronic disease… and chronic disease come from three big things- obesity, lack of exercise and smoking… and it also results in 40% of the premature deaths in the United States…." (http://www.cnn.com/2009/POLITICS/06/19/sotu.cleveland.clinic/index.html?iref=newssearch) (9/29/09)

67 Studies have shown that woman who average 3 hours of strenuous exercise per week reduce the risk of breast cancer by 20%. http://www.nytimes.com/2008/05/13/health/13breast.html?_r=1, (10/8/09)

68 Center for Disease Control, January 2010.

69 Medline Plus, " Heart disease in women", NIH: National Heart, Lung and Blood Institute, http://www.nlm.nih.gov/medlineplus/heartdiseaseinwomen.html, (6/26/2011)

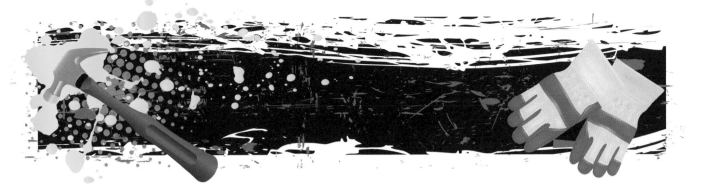

Chapter Four

Transitioning to a Lifestyle of Optimal Health

An important part of attaining and maintaining optimal health is to build healthy nutrition and fitness into a lifestyle so your appetite prefers healthier foods and your body prefers exercise.

The key ingredient to transition to healthy nutrition is to make gradual yet significant changes to your eating habits.

Over the years I have eaten hot dogs, potato chips and drank at least one soda while watching a sporting event or a favorite TV show. Considering how long I had been eating in this manner, it would have been difficult for me to immediately replace this meal with two carrot sticks, three celery sticks and a glass of carrot juice. Such a draconian change would make it difficult for me to consistently eat healthier meals over a long period of time. Instead, I made gradual yet significant changes by substituting healthy foods for unhealthy foods. I transitioned to a healthier meal by substituting the regular hot dog (180 calories and 13 grams of fat)[70] for a 97% fat free hot dog (that typically contains 40 calories and 1.5 grams of fat). I also replaced regular potato chips with tasty substitutes such vegetable chips, organic potato chips, or all-natural oven-baked sweet potato fries. I had to wean myself off of soft drinks and "fruit" drinks, which often contain a prodigious amount of sugar and various members of THE 7. Because I had been drinking soft drinks and "fruit" drinks for many years, I had to put my palate Under Construction. I went from consuming a soft drink every lunch (or dinner) to one every other meal for a four-week period. After the fourth week, I had a soft drink every third lunch for a four-week period. During the Under Construction process, I substituted soft drinks with water, all-natural sparkling water with fruit juice, and fruit juice with no added sugar. I continued the Under Construction process until it was no longer necessary for me to have soft drinks. Making these kinds of gradual changes empowered me to have healthier foods and beverages over a longer period of time, thus making my healthy eating habits a lifestyle.

Many of us have spent most of our lives eating less-than-healthy meals and snacks and consuming less-than-healthy beverages that provide little to no nutritional value to our bodies. Just as it has taken

---

70 Soar Copyright ©1995-2000, "Information about hot dogs", Recipe Source, http://www.recepesource.com/misc/hints/hot-dog-info01.html, (9/15/08)

time for us to develop less- than-healthy eating habits, it takes time to develop healthier eating habits. So, don't "bite off more than you can chew". Be patient with yourself as you are Under Construction.

Key ingredients to transition to a lifestyle of fitness include fighting through the couch potato syndrome, maintaining a consistent fitness regimen, performing the Fitness Adventure in segments, and increasing your daily physical activities.

Despite a consistent fitness regimen, I am often tempted to give into the couch potato syndrome. My 40+ year-old body feels like going home, having a late-night meal and either sitting on the couch or immediately going to sleep. However, it's imperative that I fight through these feelings. One way is to avoid thinking about the series of exercises. Instead, focus only on starting the first exercise, the interval treadmill run. You will be amazed at how starting your first exercise and working up a nice sweat will give you the physical and psychological boost to complete a Segment 1 or an entire Fitness Adventure. An additional means of fighting through the couch potato syndrome is to avoid making detours such as running a "quick" errand or stopping for a "quick" coffee before your Fitness Adventure. Detours can easily take longer than one anticipates and lead to procrastination. Instead, start your Fitness Adventure at the scheduled time. I've discovered that when I start my Fitness Adventure at the scheduled time, it often results in some of my most productive workouts. As you push through the exercise apathy, your body will reach the ultimate fitness apogee as your body actually prefers to workout. At this point, your fitness regimen has become a lifestyle.

To maintain a consistent fitness regimen, it's important to establish one that becomes an integral part of your regular schedule and not one that merely fits in your schedule. A fitness regimen that fits in your schedule is easily negotiable. If it doesn't fit you'll simply skip it. However, a fitness regimen that is an integral part of your regular schedule is non-negotiable. Whether it's arriving at the station at a particular time to take the train to the office or scheduling a particular time to drive to avoid the morning traffic, most of us develop and maintain schedules. Your health is just as important.

There are many ways to make a Day One, Day Two and Day Three Fitness Adventure an integral part of your weekly schedule. If you go to work at 9 a.m. and you are a morning person you may want to exercise before work. This may not only get you energized for the day, but will avoid any impediments to your Fitness Adventure.

You may have a work schedule that allows you to perform a split workout. For example, you can complete a portion of the Fitness Adventure during lunch and the remaining portion before work or after work. If these options do not work, then perform your Fitness Adventure after work. However, when scheduling your after work Fitness Adventure, it's imperative that you don't make detours. Instead, immediately get started. Starting quickly will leave little room for excuses or impediments.

To develop your fitness regimen into a lifestyle, it may be helpful to perform the Day One, Day Two and Day Three Fitness Adventure in segments. Use the first 12 weeks to perform Segment 1 exercises. For example, the Segment 1 of a Day Two Fitness Adventure includes an interval treadmill run, *V-PAK* I, and Tour de Burn (See BUC Fitness Adventure Chart in Appendix 3). Following the Segment 1 exercises, perform a Home Stretch. During the 12-week period, focus on developing proper form and technique as higher reps and faster speed will be attained over a period of time. Beginning the 13th week, add one additional exercise. After 12 weeks of performing Segment 1, add the *V-PAK II* starting the 13th week. Perform these exercises for 12 weeks, including a Home Stretch. Continue this process for each subsequent 12-week period until you are able to complete an entire Day One, Day Two or Day Three Fitness Adventure. Segments are an integral part of the Under Construction process that gets your body and mind accustomed to performing a consistent fitness regimen. Segments, when fully implemented, can be an important building block in your Fitness Adventure becoming a lifestyle.

Then there is making fitness a lifestyle through small yet significant daily physical activity. Like many of you, I spend most of my day sitting. During my 4:34 a.m. train ride into the city, I'm sitting for approximately 60 minutes. I then sit during my 10-minute bus ride from the train station to the office building. Once I get into the office at 6 a.m., I spend most of my day sitting at a desk. By 5 p.m., I leave the office and I do more sitting on the way home. Some research has shown that excessive sitting can contribute to obesity and other physical ailments[71].

To offset the adverse physical effects of excessive sitting, I implement small yet significant forms of calorie-burning physical activity. For example, to avoid simply sitting at my desk most of the day I stand when making a call to or hosting a conference call with a client. I set the alarm on my phone that chimes periodically throughout the day as a reminder to stand or walk across the office. When I have to go to the rest room, located at the opposite end of the office floor, I take a brisk walk or slow jog. If you are drinking at least 64 ounces of water throughout the day, you may find yourself jogging to the restroom out of necessity. I also walk to get my lunch instead of having it delivered. Two to three times per week, during off-workout days, I take the stairs when going to and returning from lunch. Taking the stairs to and from the office ignites the body's ability to burn calories. If you are located on a high floor, use the Under Construction process to build endurance. If you are located on the 10th floor, start by walking down 2-3 flights then take the elevator to the ground floor. When returning to the office, walk up 2-3 flights, and then take the elevator to your office floor. As you continue to build endurance, add a flight of stairs to your trip.

I have changed the way I travel to and from the office. Instead of sitting for 10 minutes on the bus ride between the train station and the office building, I take a 15-minute walk each way. Two or three times per week, I stand during my train ride home. I used the Under Construction process to get my body accustomed to standing during the train ride. When I first started standing on the train it was for the first 2-3 stops, and then I'd sit down for most of the stops and then stand again for the last 2-3 train stops. Over time, I continued to stand one additional train stop until I was able to stand for an entire ride home.

During the weekends, you can perform various physical activities to burn calories. In the summer, I wash the family vehicles and in the winter I plow the snow around our home following a typical Chicago snow storm. As I'm working, I periodically contract my abs, holding each contraction

---

71   Elin Ekblom-Bak, "Are we facing a new paradigm of inactivity physiology", British Journal of Sports Medicine, http://bjsm.bmj.com/content/44/12/834, (2/4/2010).

for 10-20 seconds. I not only save the money that would be used to pay for such services, but I spark calorie-burning and define my abs.

Building healthy nutrition and fitness into a lifestyle can assist in reducing risk to cancer, heart disease and other chronic illnesses including those that result from family history. According to the Cleveland Clinic Genomic Medicine Group: "you can change behaviors that affect your health, such as smoking, inactivity, and poor eating habits. People with family history of chronic disease may have the most to gain from making lifestyle changes. In many cases, making these changes can reduce your risk of disease even if the disease runs in your family."[72]

---

72 Cleveland Clinic Genomic Medicine, "The importance of knowing your family history"; The Cleveland Clinic © 1995-2010; www.my.clevelandclinic.org, (7/24/10).

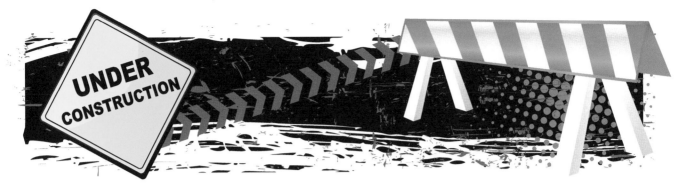

Chapter Five
"Know When To Fold Em"
&
Celebrate with Junk Food

A s we age, it becomes equally important for us to "know when to fold em," giving the body the rest it needs and deserves. Resting allows your muscles time to heal and reduces the risk of muscle strain. Take 1-2 days of rest between Day One, Day Two and Day Three Fitness Adventures so your muscles can heal. Soak your body in a jacuzzi at least once a month to provide your muscles relief. If you do not have access to a jacuzzi, fill your bath tub with warm water and add Epson or lavender bath salt. Epson Salt reduces inflammation to relieve muscle cramps, promotes muscle relaxation and assists muscles in functioning properly[73]. Lavender-based bath salts produce a lavender aroma which some studies have shown can contribute to relaxing the entire body[74]. Most importantly, attempt to consistently get 7-8 hours of sleep per night. Getting less sleep than the body needs can increase the risk of feeling too tired to exercise, consuming food in an attempt to counter drowsiness, and/or eating higher calorie and high fat foods[75]. According to a study conducted by the University Of Chicago Medical Center, a lack of sleep can contribute to increased risk of hypertension and obesity[76]. To assure that I get 7-8 hours of sleep per night, I set my cell phone to chime approximately 1 hour before bed time. This serves as a reminder to begin to wind down and prepare for sleep. I also keep the room cool[77] and reduce the amount of light in the room by shutting off the TV and cell phone, drawing the curtains close and turning my digital clock toward the wall to reduce the neon-like glow.

73 Epson Salt Industry Council, "Health benefits", http://www.epsomsaltcouncil.org/health-benefits.htm (10/9/2008)

74 Laura Johannes, " A scent to lull you to sleep", Wall Street Journal/Health, www.WSJ.com, (8/24/2010)

75 St-Onge MP, "Short sleep duration increase energy intake but does not change energy expenditure in normal-weight individuals", New York Obesity Research Center, http://www.ncbi.nlm.nih.gov/pubmed, (Aug. 2011)

76 University of Chicago Medical Center (10/21/1999), "Lack of sleep alters hormones, metabolism, stimulates effects of aging, University of Chicago, http://wwwuchospitals.edu/news/1999/19991021-sleepdebt.html, (3/2/2009)

77 Onen SH, "Prevention and treatment of sleep disorders through regulation of sleeping habits", Clinique du Sommeil, CHRU, Lille, http://www.ncbi.nlm.nih.gov/pubmed, (3/12/1994)

It's also important to reward the body for weight goals attained. At 40+ year old, I weigh myself once a week, on Sunday morning. Whenever I attain weight goals, I celebrate. For example, one weight goal that I set at 40+ years old was to return to the weight I maintained during my years as an undergraduate at the University of Hartford. When I attained this goal, I celebrated by treating myself to junk food. I go to a fast food restaurant, order a single burger with fries and a soda. However, even during these times of celebration I take certain precautions. First, I complete a pre-celebration workout: A 5-minute moderate speed treadmill run, 5 minutes of jumping rope, and a 5-minute moderate speed ride on a stationary bike (or a bike attached to a cycle trainer) with little to no rest between each exercise. The primary purpose of the pre-celebration exercises is to get the body's calorie-burning metabolism revved up before the meal. Secondly, I alter my fast food order. I do not "Super Size" or "Biggie" my fries or soda. I even request the cup be filled with as much ice as possible so that I am actually getting less soda. I order my burger plain, which helps me avoid fixings that are typically high in saturated fat and calories such as creamy sauces, mayonnaise, etc. I take the entire meal home and apply fixings such as:

- Organic or all-natural mustard
- Organic ketchup
- Avocado slices or guacamole
- Dark leafy vegetable
- Organic or 2% milk cheese

5 to 10 minutes after the meal, I perform a post-celebration workout: A 5-minute moderate speed bike ride on a stationary bike, 5 minutes of jumping rope, and a 5-minute moderate speed treadmill run with little to no rest between each exercise. The purpose of the post-celebration workout is to rev up the body's calorie-burning metabolism following the celebration.

However, do not celebrate with junk food each time you attain a weight goal. Find other means of celebrating such as treating yourself to a major sporting event, massage, shopping spree, or trip out of town. Whatever the celebration, give yourself various rewards for attaining your weight goals. You deserve it.

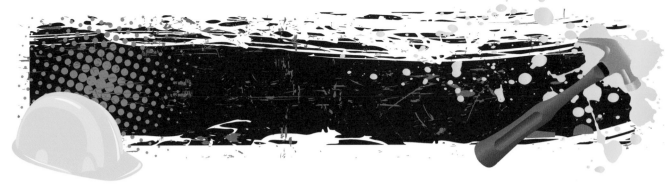

Chapter Six

The Next Level

As you develop your Fitness Adventure, some of the exercises described in the previous chapters may be challenging while others may be less-than challenging. If you find that it's difficult to complete a certain number of reps for a given exercise, don't get discouraged. Simply do a number of reps that are attainable. If you are a fitness neophyte performing a particular exercise using weights, start at a weight level that is manageable.

What's important with regards to these exercises is the use of proper form and technique. For example, with chin/pull-ups, it may be necessary for you to start with a lower number of reps to assure that you are using the proper form and technique.

If the exercises are not challenging enough, increase the number of reps and/or amount of weight. Once you've maxed out the number of reps or weight levels while maintaining proper form and technique, you can take your Fitness Adventure to The Next Level.

Next Level exercises are advanced versions of some of the exercises described in Chapter Three. These exercises can be used as substitutes for Fitness Adventure exercises that are (or have become over time) less challenging. Next Level exercises will not only burn calories and further develop strength and endurance, but also will make your Fitness Adventure even more adventurous.

Push-ups-NL (strengthens core and tones chest, biceps, and triceps):

- Plyo push-up: Get into a standard push-up position with arms at shoulders width and contract your abs. This is the starting position (fig. 51). While contracting your abs, take 3 seconds to lower your body until your elbows are at a 90-degree angle (fig. 52). Then explode upward raising your torso off the floor and clap your hands mid air (fig. 53). That is one rep.

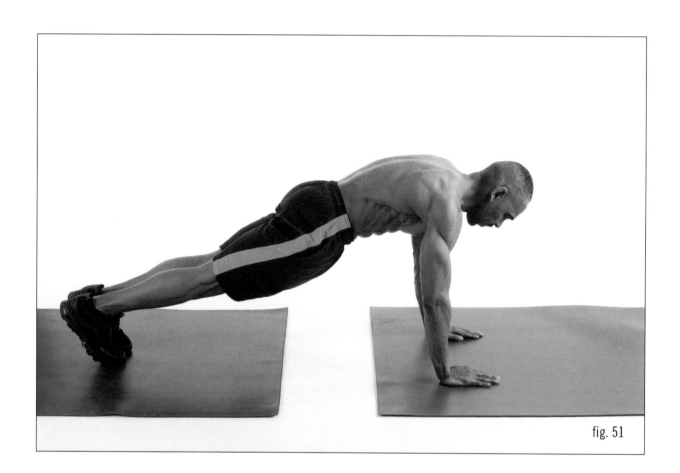

fig. 51

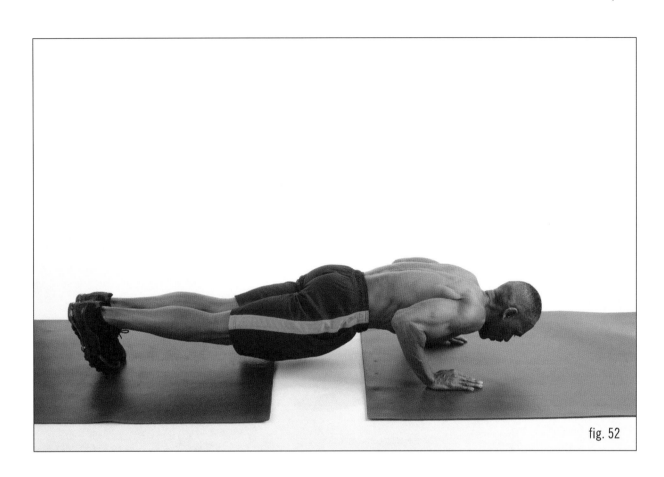

fig. 52

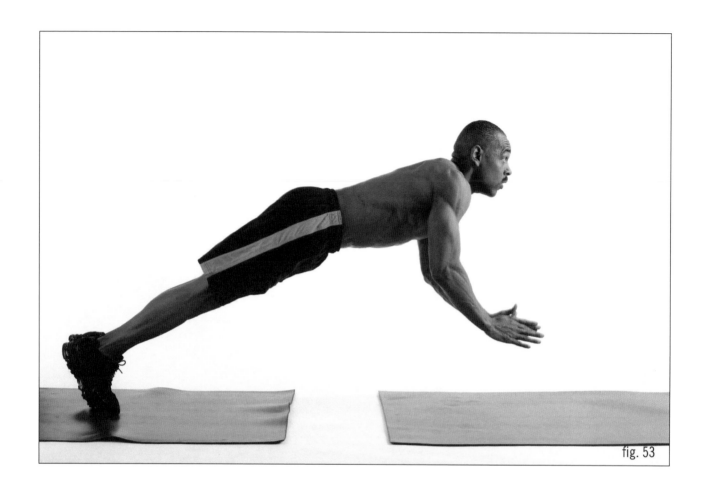

fig. 53

- Bosu plyo push-up: Get into a push-up position. However, place your hands on the top center of the Bosu and extend your legs behind you at shoulders width. This is the starting position (fig. 54). Similar to the plyo push-up, lower your body until your elbows are at a 90-degree angle, then explode upward and clap your hands midair (fig. 55). Land with your left hand on the ball and your right hand on the floor (fig. 56). From this position, explode up, clap midair, and land with your right hand on the ball and your left hand on the floor. That is one rep.

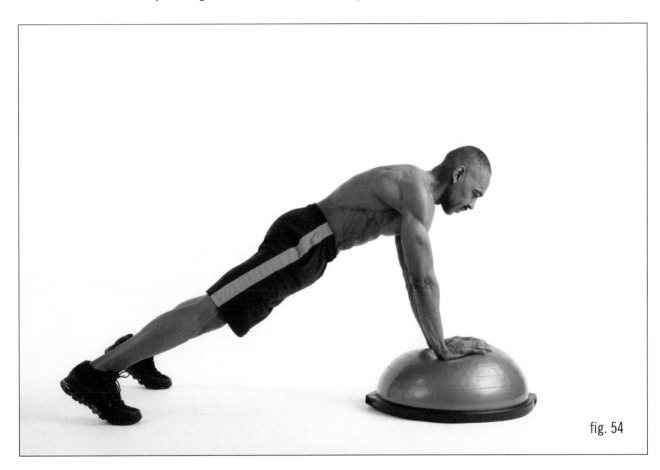

fig. 54

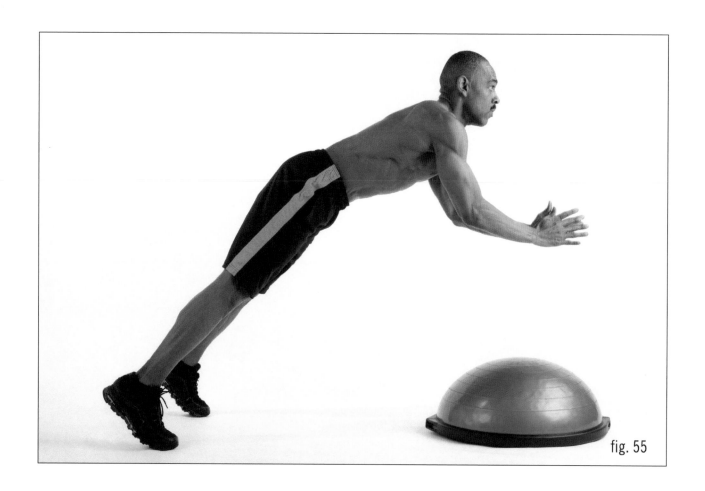

fig. 55

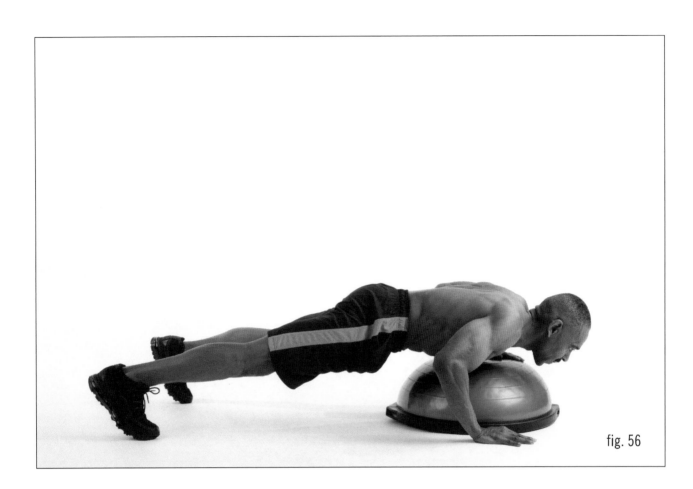

fig. 56

- Wide-arm Bosu push-up: Place the Bosu on the domed side and get into a standard push-up position with hands holding the edges of the ball. This is the starting position (fig. 57). While contracting your abs, take 3 seconds to lower your body until your elbows are at a 90-degree angle (fig. 58). Pause for 1 second. Then take 1 second to raise your body to the starting position. That is one rep. Once you've maxed out the number of reps, take it to the Next Level (and further strengthen your core) by placing a racquet (or tennis) ball in the valve inlet located in the center of the flat side of the Bosu and your shins and tops of your feet along the top of a stability ball (See fig. 41). As you perform the exercise, keep the Bosu leveled to avoid the racquetball rolling out of the inlet. Do not stop the exercise if the ball rolls out. Aim to maintain better balance to keep the racquetball in the inlet during subsequent reps.

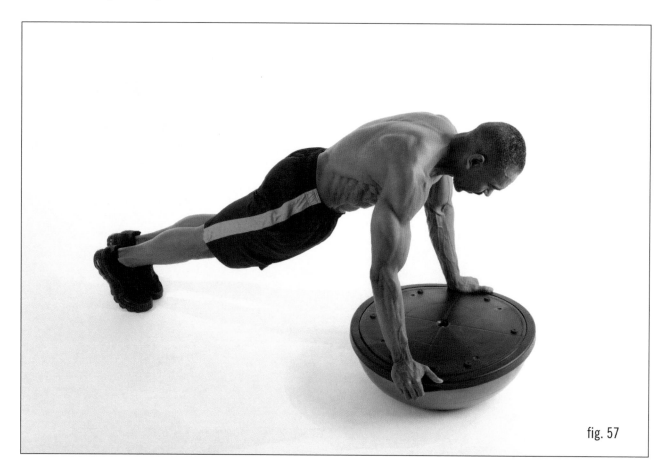

fig. 57

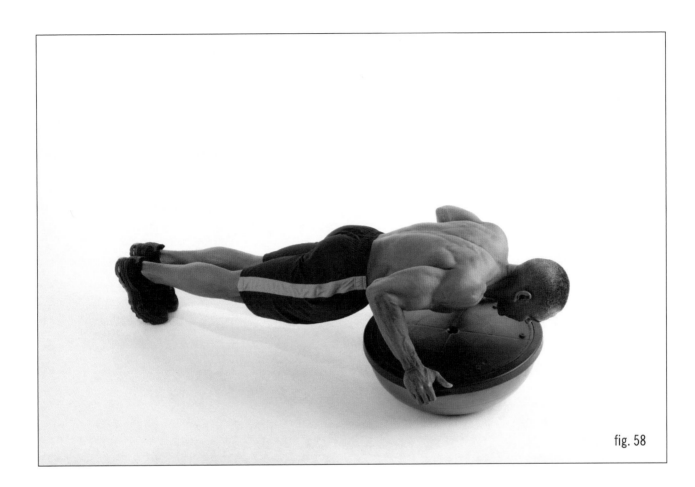

fig. 58

- Stability ball with Bosu push-up: Similar to a stability ball push-up, place your hands on the upper sides of the stability ball. However, place your feet on the domed side of a Bosu. This is the starting position (fig. 59). While contracting your abs, take 3 seconds to lower your body until your elbows are at a 90-degree angle (fig. 60). Pause for 1 second. Then take 1 second to raise your body to the starting position. That is one rep.

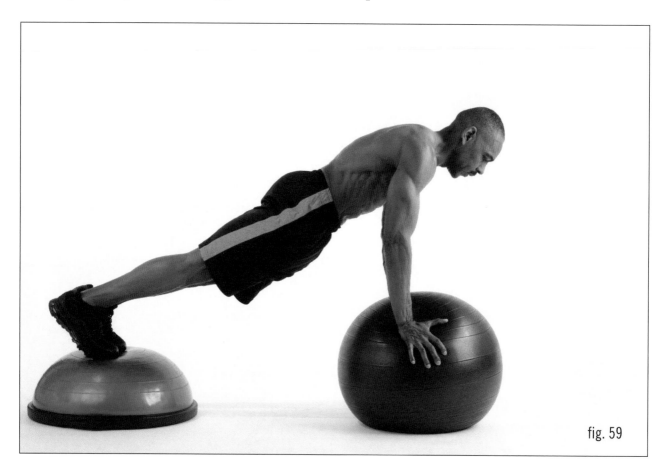

fig. 59

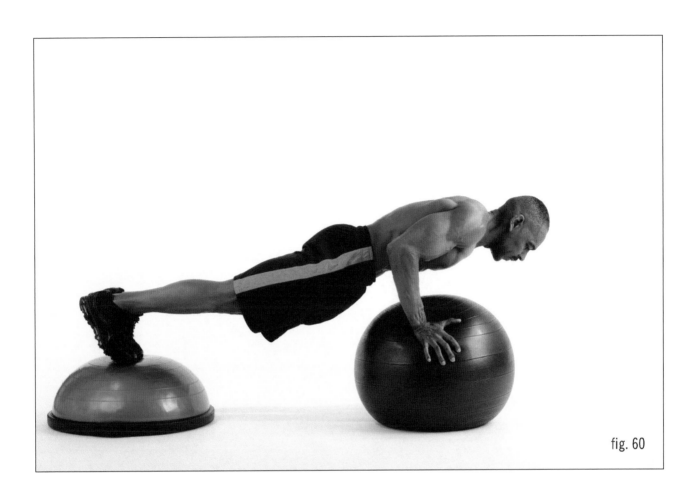

fig. 60

❧ **Crunches and Planks- NL (strengthens core and tones abs)**

- Running crunch: Sit on your buttocks and lean back until your abs are fully contracted. With legs in mid-air and knees slightly bent, balance yourself on the space between your buttocks and tail bone. From this position, raise your right knee while swinging your left arm upward then raise your left knee while swinging your right arm upward. That is one rep. During the exercise, your arms and legs should be moving as if you are running.

- Bosu ball running crunch: Sit on the domed (inflatable) side of the Bosu and lean back until your abs are fully contracted. With legs in mid-air and knees slightly bent, balance yourself on the space between your buttocks and tail bone (fig. 61). From this position, raise your right knee while swinging your left arm (fig. 62) then raise your left knee while swinging your right arm. That is one rep. During the exercise, your arms and legs should be moving as if you are running.

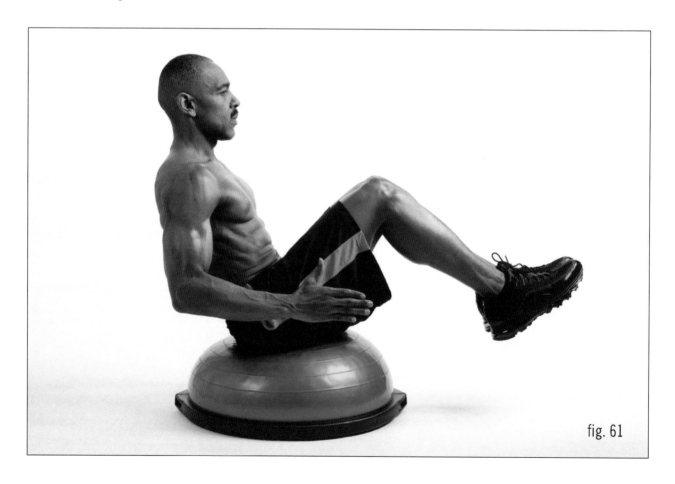

fig. 61

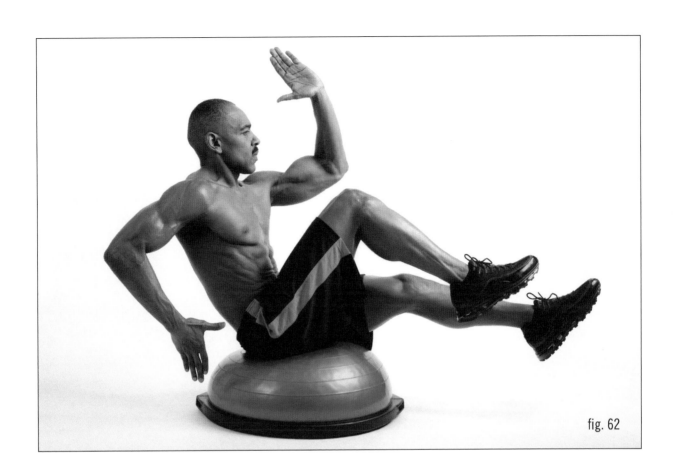

fig. 62

- Stability ball crunch with strength training ball: Sit on a stability ball with legs shoulders width apart and knees at a 90-degree angle. While holding a strength training (or medicine) ball above your head, lean back to a position that is slightly greater than a 90-degree angle to maintain tension on your abs. This is the starting position (fig. 63). While contracting your abs and holding the strength training ball over head, take 3 seconds to lean back until your back is on the ball (fig. 64) and 3 seconds to raise your upper torso to the starting position. That is one rep. To further strengthen your oblique muscles, you can add a twisting motion. From the lower position (when your back is on the ball) raise your upper torso to the right (See fig. 40). Then return to the lower position, and then raise your upper torso to the left. That is one rep. Using a strength training ball while performing this exercise makes it more difficult to maintain balance which further strengths your core and other muscles. When performing exercises using a strength training ball, start with a 2-lb ball to maintain proper form and technique. As you build strength and endurance, increase the number of reps and /or the weight of the strength training ball accordingly.

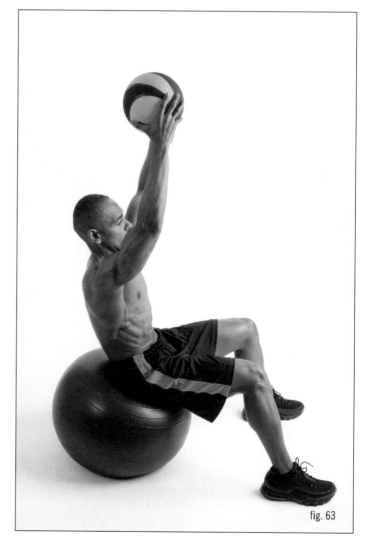

fig. 63

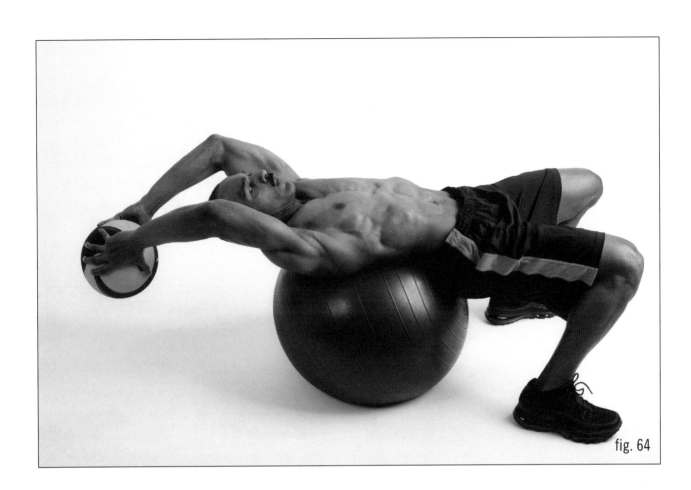

fig. 64

- Stability ball crunch toss and catch: Similar to the stability ball crunch with strength training ball, sit on a stability ball with legs at shoulders width and knees at a 90-degree angle. While holding a strength training ball above your head, lean back to a position that is slightly greater than a 90-degree angle to maintain tension on your abs. This is the starting position (See fig. 63). While contracting your abs, take 3 seconds to lean back until your back is on the ball (See fig. 64). As you raise your upper torso to the starting position, toss the ball above your head (fig. 65) and catch it. That is one rep. Tossing and catching the ball increases the difficulty of maintaining balance which strengthens your core and other muscles.

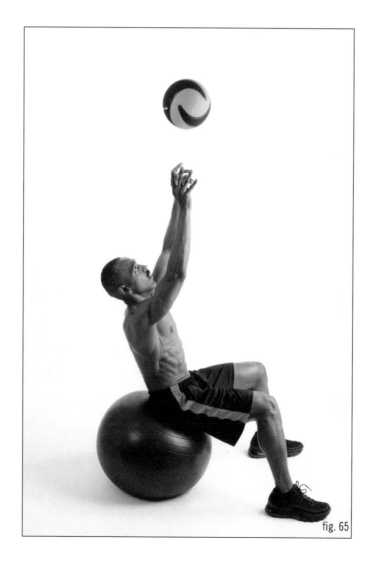

fig. 65

- Hanging leg raise: Similar to hanging knee raises, place each arm in an ab strap (your arms should be positioned at shoulders width) so that your body is supported by your arms and shoulders. Hold the top of the ab straps with your hands and contract your abs. Your body should be hanging from the ab straps with your feet off the floor. This is the starting position (See fig. 21). While contracting your abs, take 1 second to raise your knees to your chest (See fig. 22), pause for 1 second, then take 3 seconds to lower your legs to the starting position then immediately raise your legs to the left until your feet are above your left hand (fig. 66) and pause for 1 second. Return to the starting position. Then immediately raise knees to your chest holding the position for 1 second, return to the starting position then immediately raise your legs to the right until your feet are above your right hand and pause for 1 second. Return to the starting position. That is one rep.

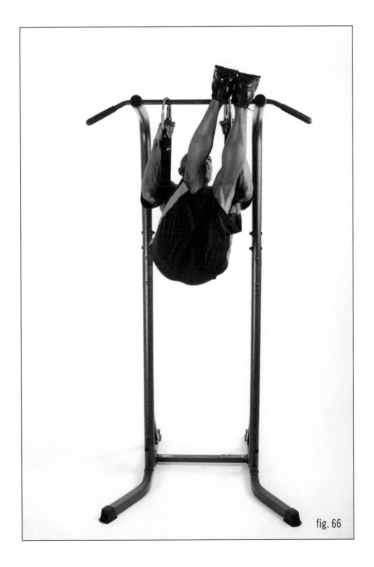

fig. 66

- Stability ball plank with Bosu: Get into a plank position, but instead of resting your forearms on the floor, rest your forearms on the top of the stability ball while resting your feet on the domed side of Bosu (fig. 67). Once you are able to hold the plank for 2 minutes, try holding the plank with your eyes closed.

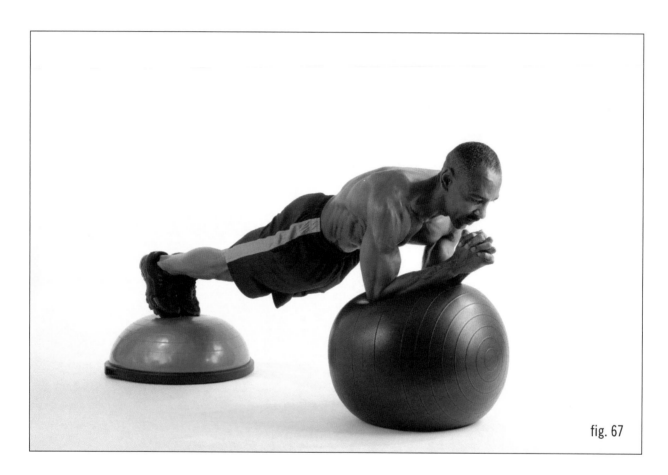

fig. 67

🦐 Pull/Chin-up-NL (tones abs and strengthens arm and back muscles)

- Pull-up-knee-raise: Similar to the pull-up exercise, position your hands on the chin-up bar slightly wider than shoulders width, your palms facing away from your body, and contract your abs. Your body should be hanging with your feet off the floor. This is the starting position (fig. 68). While contracting your abs, take 1 second to raise your body until your chin is above the bar (fig. 69). Hold this position and raise your knees toward your chest (fig. 70). Then lower your knees while keeping your chin above the bar (See fig. 69). Then take 3 seconds to lower your body to the starting position. That is one rep.

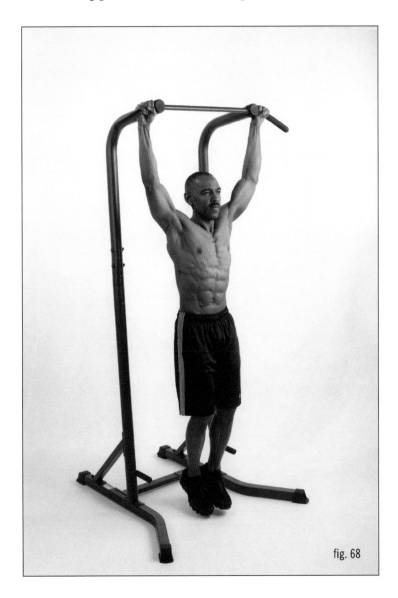

fig. 68

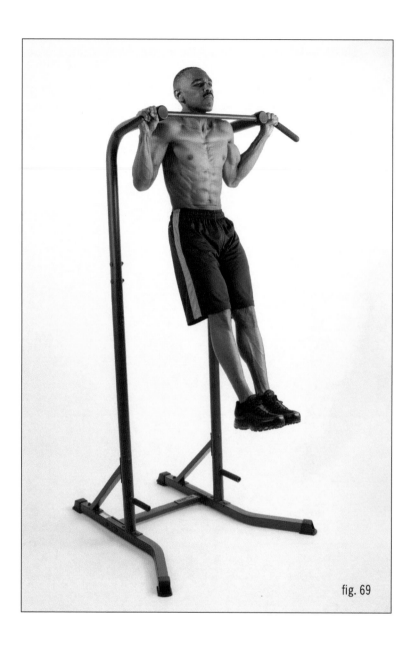

fig. 69

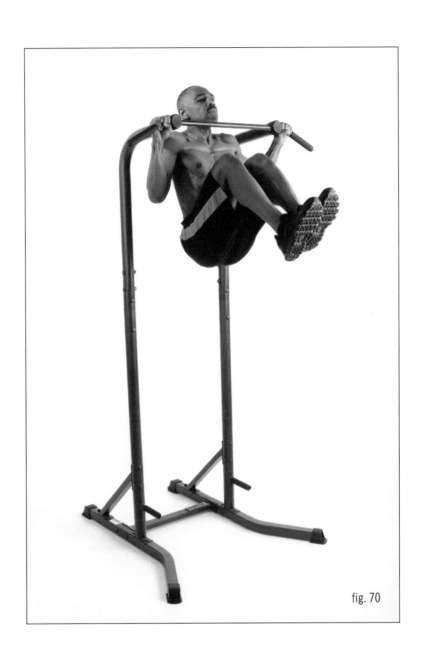

fig. 70

- Pull-up-push-off: Similar to the pull-up exercise, position your hands slightly wider than shoulders width, your palms facing away from your body, and contract your abs. Your body should be hanging with your feet off the floor. This is the starting position (See fig. 68). While contracting your abs, take 1 second to raise your body until your chin is above the bar (See fig. 69). Pause for 1 second. As you slowly lower your body, push your body away from the bar (fig. 71) while returning to the starting position. This is one rep.

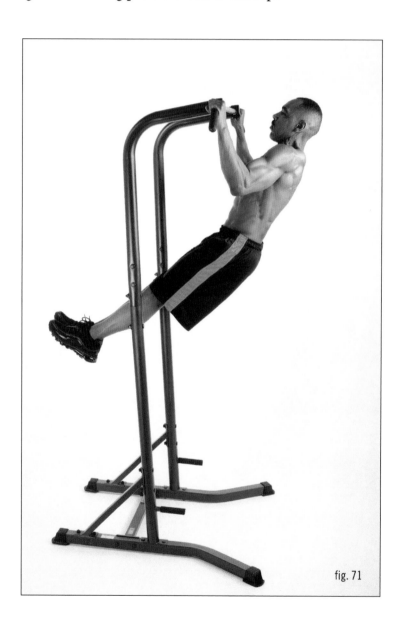

fig. 71

- 1 ½ Chin-up: Using a chin-up bar, get into a chin-up position with your hands slightly within shoulders width, your palms facing your body, and contract your abs. Your body should be hanging with your feet off the floor. This is the starting position (fig. 72). While contracting your abs, raise your body half way (fig. 73). Pause for 1 second. Then lower your body to the starting position. Then immediately raise your body until your chin is above the bar (fig. 74). Pause for 1 second. Then take 3 seconds to lower your body to the starting position. That is one rep. The ½ chin up motion during the exercise benefits the biceps (the large muscle at the upper front portion of the arm) while the full chin-up motion benefits the Latissimus dorsi (or "lats") muscles located along the middle/lower portion of the back.

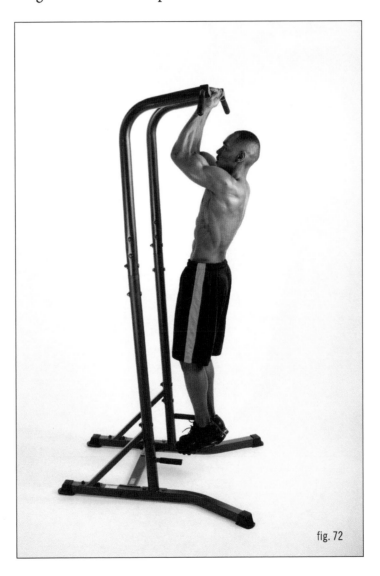

fig. 72

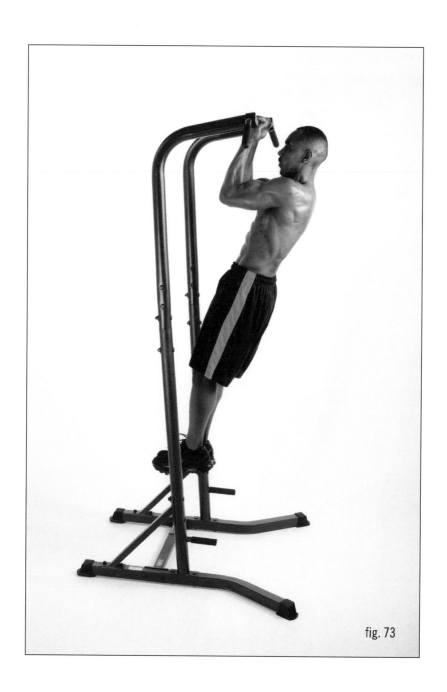

fig. 73

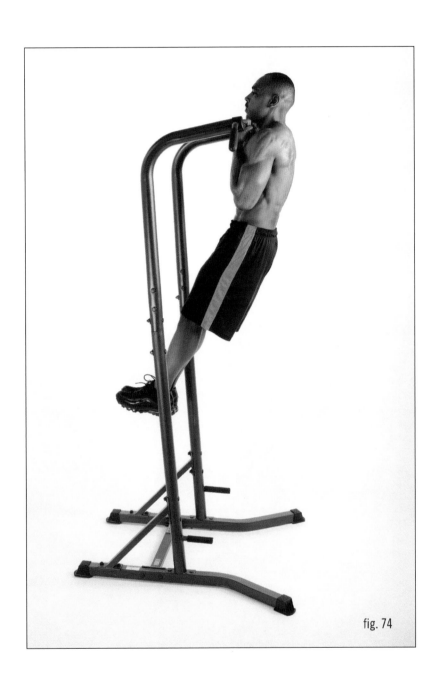

fig. 74

Body weight squat-NL (tones entire body, particularly leg muscles)

- 1 ½ Bosu body weight squat with strength training ball: Stand on the domed side of a Bosu ball with feet with in shoulders width, slightly bend your knees and contract your abs while holding a strength training ball out and in front of your chest. This is the starting position (fig. 75). Keeping your back slightly arched and abs contracted lower your body until your knees are at a 90-degree angle (fig. 76) then raise your body half way while simultaneously lifting the ball out and in front of your chest. (fig. 77). Then immediately return to the lower position with knees at a 90-degree angle (See fig. 76). Then immediately raise yourself to the starting position. That is one rep.

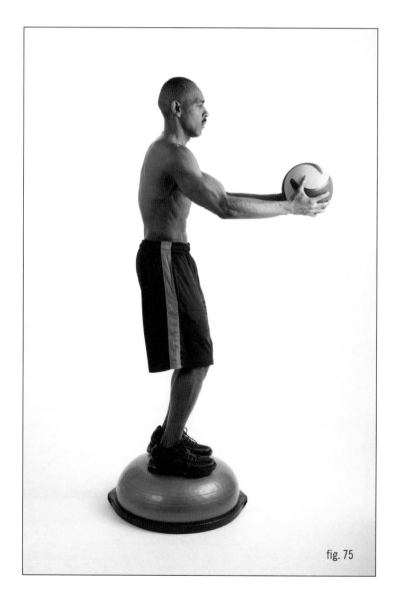

fig. 75

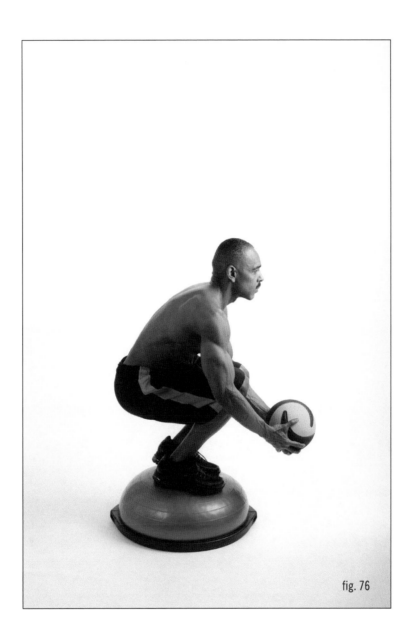

fig. 76

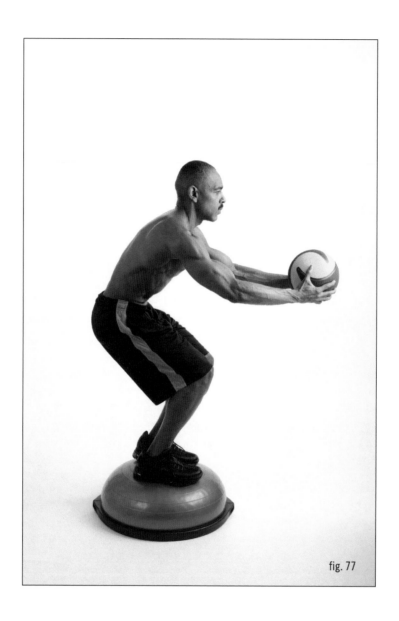

fig. 77

- 1 ½ Bosu body weight squat toss and catch: Similar to the 1 ½ Bosu body weight squat with strength training ball, stand on the domed side of a Bosu ball with feet with in shoulders width. While holding a strength training ball out and in front of your chest, slightly bend your knees and contract your abs. This is the starting position (See fig. 75). Keeping your back slightly arched and abs contracted, lower your body until your knees are at a 90-degree angle (See fig. 76), then raise your body half way while simultaneously tossing and catching the ball (with your finger tips) out and in front of your chest (See fig. 77), then immediately return to the lower position. As you raise your body to the starting position, toss the ball in the air (fig. 78) and catch it. That is one rep.

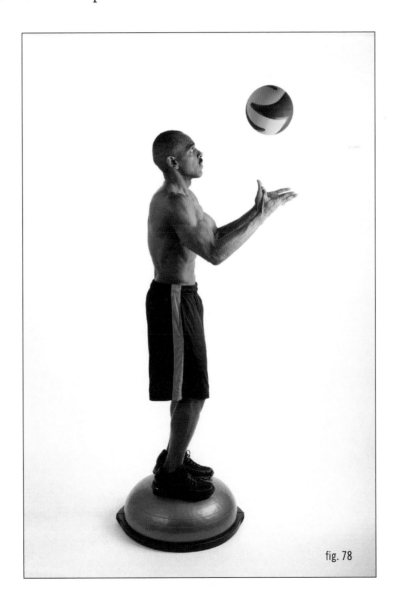

fig. 78

- 1 ½ Bosu body weight squat-flat side: To perform this exercise you must mount the Bosu ball. First place the Bosu on the domed side. While holding the Bosu in place with both hands, place your left foot approximately 1-2 inches from the left edge. (fig. 79). Then place your right foot approximately 1-2 inches from the right edge (fig. 80). Stand with your knees slightly bent. Perform the 1 ½ Bosu body weight squats as described in Chapter 3. Alternatively, you can perform the 1 ½ Bosu body weight squat while holding or tossing and catching the strength training ball as previously described (See fig. 81 and fig. 82 for mounting Bosu with strength training ball). Upon completing the exercise, dismount the Bosu by holding it in place with both hands and removing your right foot followed by your left foot. Once you've maxed out the number of reps, take it to the Next Level (and further strengthen your core) by performing the exercise with a racquetball in the valve inlet as previously described.

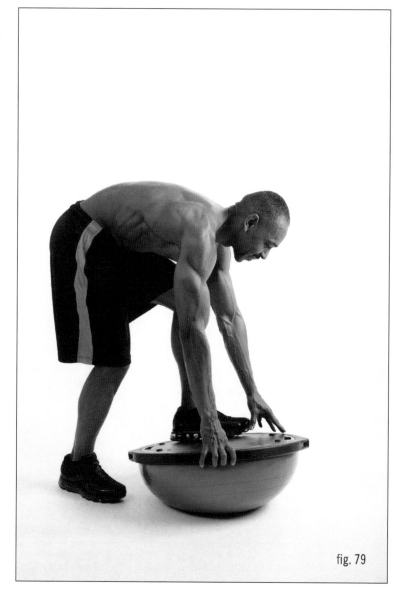

fig. 79

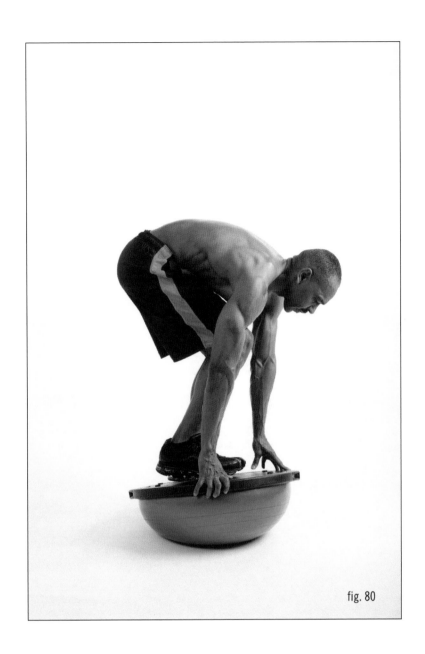

fig. 80

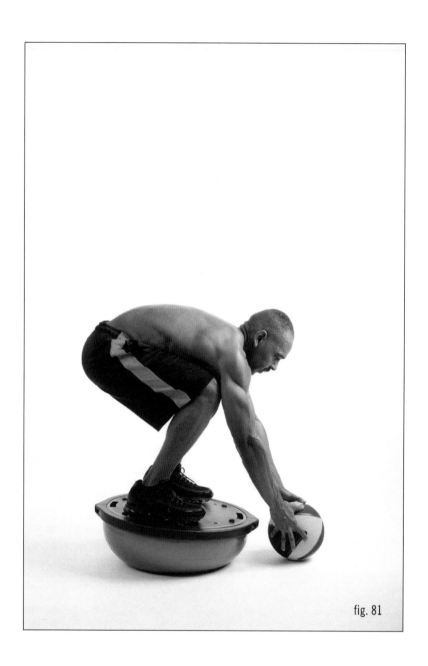

fig. 81

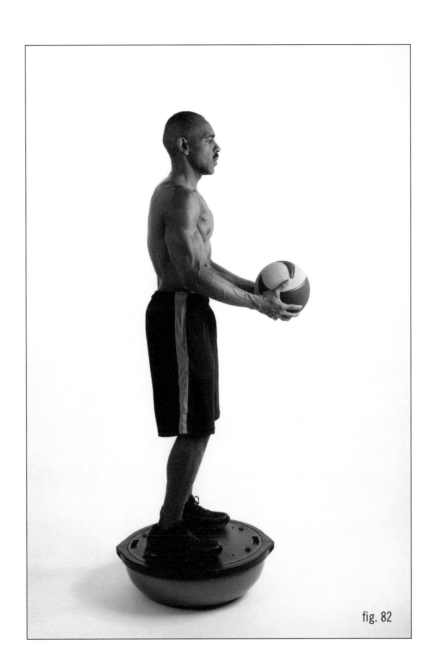

fig. 82

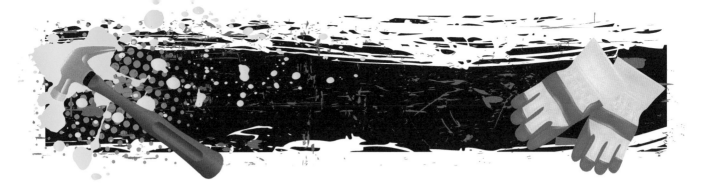

Chapter Seven

"On the Road Again"

Check the "Extra Luggage"

As an itinerate salesman, I spend a good portion of my time traveling for business purposes. Unfortunately, my 40+ year old body often pays the traveling expense through less-than-healthy airport snacks, fat-laden business meals and a lack of physical fitness during business travel. To avoid returning from a business trip with "extra luggage", weight gained during travel, I do the following:

- Pack Danger Zone and other healthy snacks: When I am waiting to take a flight, I often want a snack before I board the plane. A typical airport terminal has mostly fast food restaurants and newsstands that offer foods and snacks that contain members of THE 7 and are high in calorie and/or fat content. I often pack Danger Zone and healthy dessert snacks such as organic potato chips, vegetable chips, organic fig bars, 70% dark chocolate, and/or organic dried berries and cherries in an airtight sandwich bag. These snacks are great alternatives to the on board snacks such as crackers and cookies.

- Drink water before dinner: Drink at least two 8-ounce glasses to trick your body into feeling full, thus reducing the risk of overeating.

- Avoid soda: Drink water, cranberry juice, or fresh-squeezed lemonade. If you prefer tea, order it unsweetened and flavor it yourself to control the amount of sugar added. If you prefer alcohol, be careful because many alcohol drinks contain high calories, sugar, and carbohydrates and can easily result in you returning from a business trip with "extra luggage". For example, an 8-ounce daiquiri contains approximately 500 calories and an 8-ounce margarita contains approximately 400 calories[78]. A better alternative is red wine as it contains fewer calories than most mixed alcohol drinks and is a better antioxidant

---

78 Calorie Count, http://caloriecount.about.com/calories-daiquiri-i14010?size_grams=60.0, http://caloriecount.about.com/calories-island-oasis-margarita-i103882?size_grams=102.0, (7/28/2011)

source than white wine. However, even in the case of red wine, limit yourself to one serving as one 5-ounce glass contains approximately 120 calories[79]. For women, limiting alcohol consumption not only counters weight gain, but also can contribute to reducing the risk of breast cancer[80].

- Have a healthy, hearty appetizer: The purpose of a healthy hearty appetizer is to ruin your dinner appetite and avoid overeating during the main course. Eat appetizers that are low in fat and calories. For example, I'll eat a salad with vinaigrette dressing instead of creamy dressings such as blue cheese or Ranch. Creamy dressings are typically high in calorie and fat. I often request berries, raw nuts and/or a few strips of grilled chicken or salmon be added to my salad. The toppings not only provide my body with antioxidants, Omega-3 and protein, but also contribute to ruining my appetite before dinner is served. The heartier the salad, the better as it increases the probability of the body feeling full before the main course. Other healthy appetizers include broth, vegetable or black bean soup. However, I avoid appetizers that are high in calories or fat. Buffalo wings, previously one of my all-time favorite appetizers, contain approximately 910 calories and 81 grams of fat[81]. This is before dipping the Buffalo wings in blue cheese dressing.

- Go with mostly white meat: For my main course, I order white meats such as grilled or baked chicken or turkey breast. However, I avoid fried versions of these foods. Another healthy favorite is baked or grilled salmon which is a great source of Omega-3. Occasionally I eat steak, which is a good source of protein and iron. I order sirloin, the leanest type of steak, to keep fat content to a minimum. I also avoid smothering my steak in creamy sauces and gravy which are often high in calories and fat. I use low-calorie alternative toppings such as onions and mushrooms. I eat half the steak to avoid overeating. I compensate by filling up on vegetables such as spinach, cauliflower and/or broccoli. However, avoid drowning your vegetables in creamy sauces (See the BUC Check the "Extra Luggage" Nutrition Chart in Appendix 4).

- Back away from the rolls: I was a "carboholic" when it came to warm-buttered-white rolls. I couldn't eat enough of them. Given my love for this refined carbohydrate food, I knew going cold turkey would not be sustainable over a long period of time. As a result, I made two significant changes: I stopped adding butter to the roll and instead used olive oil which contains monounsaturated and polyunsaturated fats; secondly: I put myself Under Construction. I set up a process by which I reduced the number of rolls I ate over a certain number of

79 Joy Bauer, "Raise a glass! Wine's health benefits", MSNBC, http://www.msnbc.msn.com/id/21478144/print/1/display-mode/1098/, (6/4/2008)

80 Roni Caryn Rabin, "Reducing your risk for breast cancer, NY Times (5/13/08), http://www.nytimes.com/2008/05/13/health/13breast.html?_r=1, (10/8/09)

81 Daily Plate, "Home made buffalo wings", ©2009 Daily Plate LLC/Helping you eat smarter, http://www.thedailyplate.com/nutrition-calories/food/generic/homemade-buffalo-wings, (3/2/2009)

business trips. What assisted me in the process was drinking at least two glasses of water and eating a salad to make my body feel full, thus limiting the number of rolls I desired. Because of this process, my body no longer needs bread or rolls for my business dinner to feel complete.

⫶ Beware of the Double Ds: Dangerous Desserts are high in calories and fat. Although I typically satisfy my sweet tooth with desserts such as dark chocolate-covered fruit or a fruit plate, there are times when Double Ds such as apple pie, carrot cake, or chocolate chip cookies, seem to whisper my name. During these times, I cut a ¼ of the pie or cake (or take 1-2 cookies) and will immediately return the remainder to the server or have the remaining portion boxed to go to give to my family. I do not allow the entire dessert to remain on my plate. Adhering to the adage "out of sight, out of mind" can be extremely helpful at reducing overindulgence.

Room Service Workout

In conjunction with developing better eating habits while on the road, I've developed a fitness regimen to assist in checking the "extra luggage". When preparing to travel, I pack a jump rope. It's light, amorphous, and fits easily into a suitcase. I also determine if the hotel has a fitness center or whether there's one in close proximity. If a facility is available, I will perform a Day One, Day Two or Day Three Fitness Adventure. If not, I implement the Room Service Workout. It consists mostly of stretches and exercises that can be done in or within close proximity to your hotel room. Before starting, perform the warm-up and dynamic stretches described in Chapter 3.

The Room Service workout exercises include:

🏃 15-minute interval outdoor run: Using a sports wristwatch to monitor the time designated for the incremental increase and decrease in speed per interval, perform a 15-minute interval run outdoors modeled after the Day One, Day Two or Day Three interval treadmill run. For example, increase and decrease speed modeled after a Day One or Day Two interval treadmill run; for two minutes perform a slow jog, the next three minutes a moderately faster jog, the next two minutes return to a slow jog, etc. You can adjust your running speed modeled after a Day Three interval treadmill run. For example, perform a slow jog for two minutes, perform a moderately fast jog for two minutes, followed by a moderately faster jog for two minutes, etc. If there are hills near your hotel, use them to replicate the inclines used during the interval treadmill run.

🏃 Burpee: This exercise strengthens and tones the entire body. Stand with your feet at shoulders width, arms at your side, and contract your abs. This is the starting position. While contracting your abs, crouch down and place the palms of your hands on the floor with your arms at shoulders width (fig. 83), then kick your feet out behind you (fig. 84). Perform a standard pushup. Return to the crouch position by bringing your knees under your chest with palms of your hands on the floor (See fig. 83). Then jump up (fig. 85). That is one rep. Perform 4 reps. After a 60-second active rest, perform 3 reps. Take a 60-second active rest.

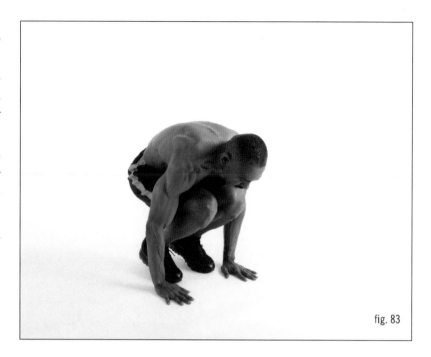

fig. 83

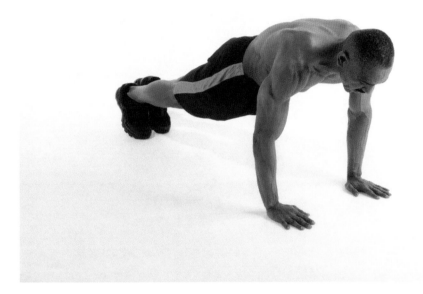

fig. 84

- Planks: Hold this position (as described in Chapter 3) for 20 seconds. After a 60-second active rest, perform another plank. Hold position for 10 seconds. Take a 60-second active rest.
- *V*-PAK V: Includes push-ups to build upper body strength and 1 ½ body weight squats to build lower body strength (See Chapter 3 for description of exercises):
    - Standard push-ups: Do 4 reps. Take a 30-second active rest.
    - 1 ½ Body weight squats: Do 6 reps. Take a 30-second active rest.
    - Close hand push-ups: Do 3 reps. Take a 30-second active rest.
    - 1 ½ Body weight squats: Do another set of body weight squats. Do 5 reps. Take a 30-second active rest.

- Feet elevated push-ups: Place your feet on a chair or on the edge of the bed so your body is at a 45-degree angle. Do 2 reps. Take a 30-second active rest.
- 1 ½ Body weight squats: Do another set of body weight squats. Do 4 reps. Take a 60-second active rest.

🏃 Bicycle crunches (as described in Chapter 3): Do 4 reps. Take a 60-second active rest. Then do 3 reps. Take a 60-second active rest.

🏃 Jump Rope: Find a location near your hotel room and jump rope for 10 minutes.

🏃 Home Stretch: Following your room service work out, perform a Home Stretch. Call room service and order an 8-ounce (or more) smoothie, chocolate milk or other refreshing drink to replenish your body following the Home Stretch.

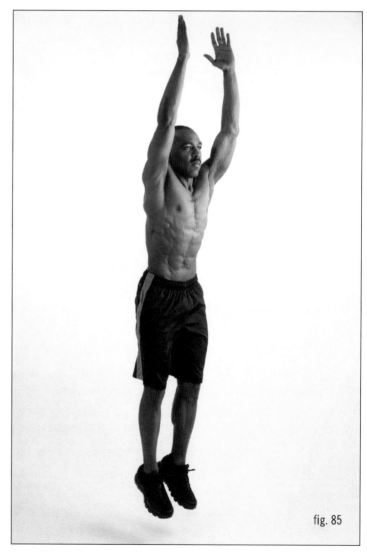

fig. 85

To keep your Room Service Workout adventurous, add 1 rep to each upper and lower body set (and 1 second to each set of planks) every 4th trip (See BUC Room Service Workout Chart in Appendix 5).

When I do not have enough time to do a Room Service Workout, I attempt to do a Workout Appetizer before dinner. The Workout Appetizer consists of:

🏃 5-minutes: Interval jump rope

🏃 5-minutes: Interval run

🏃 5-minutes: Interval (stationary) bike ride or repeat interval jump rope if a bike is not available

This series of cardio exercises serve to reignite the body's calorie-burning metabolism before dinner. I follow up dinner with the same15-minute cardio workout.

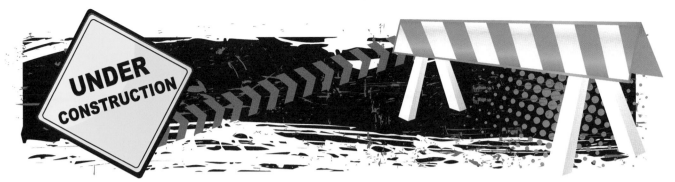

Chapter Eight

Nutrition and Fitness: A One-Two Punch Against Stress

Many of us experience stress for a variety of reasons and often suffer from the aftershocks of stress. Some are psychological, and come in the form of mental exhaustion. Other aftershocks come in the form of physical ailments, including headaches, back pain, high blood pressure and heart disease[82].

Although there are many ways of dealing with stress, many of these remedies come at the expense of health. For example, some smoke to reduce stress. Smoking maybe a temporary means of relieving stress, however, it can lead to high blood pressure, shortness of breath or cancer. Others may cope with stress by eating junk food or drinking beverages that contain large amounts of caffeine and/or sugar. These remedies can lead to weight gain. A combination of healthy nutrition and fitness can be a one-two punch against stress.

Consuming foods that contain complex carbohydrates such as fruit, vegetable, and whole grain may have a calming effect on the mind and body[83]. Fitness can play an equally critical role in reducing stress. As an equity salesman, my hours are rigorous. During my 12-plus hour day I am servicing clients and exchanging financial market information with my colleagues. I do not have a lunch hour. I run to a nearby restaurant, return to my desk and eat lunch while monitoring movements in the market via my PC. I deal with many of the job-related stress issues that you may encounter that come as a result of deadlines, multiple meetings, multi-tasking, and various technology-related glitches. If this does not make my day stressful enough, there is the ever present stress cloud that looms because of constant rumors of layoffs. During these times, the last thing many of us feel like doing is exercis-

82 Mayo Clinic Staff, "Stress Symptoms: Effects on your body, feelings and behavior", MayoClinic.com; http://www.mayoclinic.com/health/stress-symptoms/SR00008_D, (3/18/2010)

83 Daniel K. Hall-Flavin, M.D., "Generalized anxiety disorder", MayoClinic.com; http://www.mayoclinic.com/health/coping-with-anxiety/AN01589, (7/28/2011)

ing. Yet, exercise is an outstanding antidote[84]. It provides mental relief because during exercise your mind becomes more focused on movements, the use of proper form and technique while exercising, breathing regularly during reps, etc. Secondly, exercise counters stress by increasing endorphins, neurotransmitters in your brain that provide you with a sense of well being[85]. Completing an exercise or a fitness regimen can boost self-confidence, energy and provide you with a general sense of accomplishment, all of which can contribute to reducing stress.

Then there is the stress that one experiences as a result of losing a job. I lost my job in 2009. What made matters more stressful is it occurred during a time when large financial institutions were failing. That resulted in hiring freezes throughout the industry. This caused an incredible amount of stress given that I had a house mortgage, monthly car payment and my wife and three kids to support. Nevertheless, one of the antidotes that I used during this stressful time was fitness. Even when I didn't feel like it, I fought through those feelings and maintained a consistent fitness regimen. I would perform a series of exercises before job interviews. Completing these exercises not only gave me a sense of accomplishment, but gave me additional energy and confidence, intangibles needed for a successful job interview.

---

84   Mayo Clinic Staff, "Exercise: Rev up your routine to reduce stress", MayoClinic.com; http://www.mayoclinic.com/health/exercise-and-stress/SR00036, (5/18/2009)

85   Encyclopedia.com, "Endorphins", http://www.encyclopedia.com/topic/endorphins.aspx#1E1-endorphi, (3/18/2010); Mayo Clinic Staff, "Exercise: Rev up your routine to reduce stress", MayoClinic.com; http://www.mayoclinic.com/health/exercise-and-stress/SR00036, (5/18/2009)

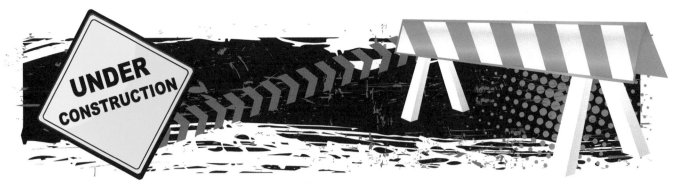

Epilogue

Body Under Construction
Tidbits

🍴 Nutritional Tidbits
- Make **gradual yet significant changes** to your eating habits
- **Read the labels**
- Avoid **THE 7**
- Drink water to **trick your body into feeling full**
- **Avoid** eating food out of **boredom**
- Utilize the **Danger Zone (DZ) Snacks** between meals and before **Big Eating Holidays**
- Go **Under Construction** to reduce consumption of soft/"fruit" drinks and refined rice/bread
- Consume more white meats like **fish, turkey and skinless chicken breast**
- Consume **organic** or **all-natural** products as often as possible
- **Ruin** your dinner appetite
- Eat **Slowly,** take a **Meal Halftime** and **After Meal Break**
- Get an **annual physical**
- Remember you are **Under Construction, so be patient with yourself**
- **Don't give up**

🏃 Fitness Tidbits
- Make your Fitness Adventure an **integral** part of your regular weekly schedule
- Set **attainable** fitness goals
- Maintain **constant movement** throughout exercises and **active rest** periods
- Focus on utilizing **proper form and technique** by reviewing exhibits of exercises every 2 weeks
- **Warm up** your body before exercise through various movements and **dynamic stretching**
- Schedule a workout around the **Big Eating Holidays**
- Perform the **Home Stretch** following each workout
- **Rest your body** 1-2 days between workouts

- **Celebrate** when weight goals are attained
- **Weigh yourself** no more than **once a week**
- Get **7-8 hours** of sleep per night
- Get an **annual physical**
- Remember you are **Under Construction, so be patient with yourself**
- **Don't give up**

**Consult your healthcare provider before commencing an exercise or nutrition program**

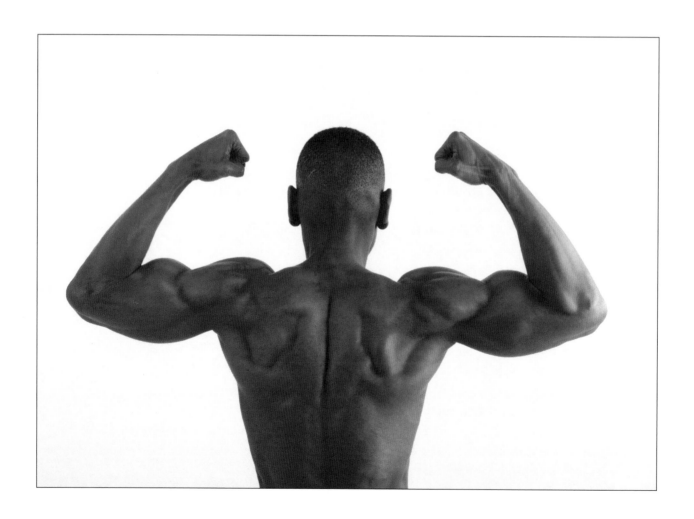

BUC
Lunch, Dinner, Dessert, and DZ Snack Recipes

The following are the recipes for suggested lunch, dinner, dessert and DZ Snack described in Chapter Two. The nutritious foods and ingredients that I use to prepare breakfast, lunch and dinner can be easily attained at specialty grocery stores that primarily sell all-natural or organic foods, within designated areas at supermarkets, or can be purchased at various online food retailers.

Lunch Recipe

Turkey Burger (4-5 patties)
Total time to prepare and cook: 30 minutes
Ingredients:

1 pound 99% lean ground turkey	1 tablespoon onion powder
1 ½ tablespoons jerk seasoning	1 fresh green bell pepper
1 tablespoon sea salt	½ teaspoon black pepper
1 tablespoon garlic powder	½ teaspoon parsley
1 tablespoon organic or all-natural Worcestershire sauce	

How to prepare:
1. Place ground turkey into a bowl.
2. Mix all ingredients into ground turkey.
3. Dice green pepper and mix into ground turkey.
4. Remove portions of ground turkey and pat into burger patty.
5. Cook in pan at low flame for approximately 15 minutes.

♪ <u>Chili with Ground Turkey (4-5 servings)</u>
Total time to prepare and cook: 50 minutes
Ingredients:

1 pound 99% lean ground turkey	1 small red bell pepper
1 15-ounce can black beans	2 tablespoons flaxseed meal
1 15-ounce can kidney beans	3 tablespoons chili powder
1 15-ounce can pinto beans	2 teaspoons cumin
1 6-ounce can tomato paste (preferably organic or all-natural)	3 cups water
1 small onion	Seasonings (season salt, garlic powder, and black pepper)

How to prepare:
1. Pour beans into an 8-quart boiling pot. Cook over a low flame.
2. Add the tomato paste, chili powder, cumin, flaxseed meal, and water.
3. Season to taste using season salt, garlic powder, and black pepper. Cover the pot and allow to simmer.
4. Brown the ground turkey in a skillet over a low flame. Stir the turkey periodically to prevent the ground turkey from burning.
5. While the ground turkey is browning, add diced onion and red bell pepper, and stir.
6. Pour cooked ground turkey into boiling pot. Cook for 45 minutes.

Dinner Recipes

<u>Salmon with Broccoli (1 serving)</u>
Total time to prepare and cook: 35 minutes
Ingredients:

1 6-ounce Wild Sockeye salmon filet	2 cups fresh or frozen broccoli
1 tablespoon canola or extra virgin olive oil	Seasoning (season salt, garlic powder, black pepper, parsley)

How to prepare:
1. Preheat oven to 375° F.
2. Wash salmon filet and pat dry. Place salmon filet in aluminum foil.
3. Pour tablespoon of olive oil on filet and season to taste. Close foil and place in small baking dish. Bake salmon filet for 35 minutes.
4. While salmon is baking, place broccoli in a steamer and steam cook over a low flame for 10 minutes. Season to taste.

♪ - Spicy

BBQ Chicken Breast (1 serving)

Total time to prepare and cook: 50 minutes

Ingredients:

1 6-ounce boneless skinless chicken breast	2 cups mixed vegetables
1 tablespoon canola or extra virgin olive oil	1 small sweet potato
1 tablespoon organic barbeque sauce	Seasonings (season salt, black pepper, garlic powder)
½ tablespoon of cinnamon	

How to prepare:

1. Preheat oven to 375° F
2. Season chicken breast to taste.
3. Pour olive oil in baking dish. Place seasoned chicken breast in baking dish. Cover and bake for 35 minutes.
4. Remove baking dish from oven and pour barbeque sauce over chicken breast. Place uncovered baking dish in oven and bake chicken breast for 10 minutes.
5. Place mix vegetables in a steamer and steam cook over a low flame for 10 minutes. Season to taste.
6. Place sweet potato in shallow baking dish and bake in oven (375°F) for 45 minutes. Once done, cut open sweet potato and sprinkle a ½ tablespoon of cinnamon inside.

) Tilapia with Bayou Sauce (4-5 servings)

Total time to prepare and cook: 50 minutes

Ingredients:

6 ¾-ounce tilapia fillets	1 small green bell pepper
1 ½ cups chicken or vegetable broth (preferably organic)	1 tablespoon cornstarch
¾ teaspoon cayenne pepper	1 10-ounce bag frozen mixed vegetables
¾ crushed red pepper	Seasoning (season salt, garlic powder, and black pepper)
1 small red bell pepper	

How to prepare:

1. Preheat oven to 375° F.
2. Place tilapia fillets in a 9 x 13 x 2-inch baking dish. Season fillets to taste with season salt, garlic powder, and black pepper. Cover fillets and bake in oven for 30 minutes.
3. To make bayou sauce, mix cornstarch, broth, cayenne and crushed red pepper in a bowl. Pour into saucepan and allow to simmer over a low flame.
4. After 30 minutes, remove baked tilapia fillets from the oven and sprinkle bag of frozen mixed vegetables on top. Cover the baking dish and bake for 10 minutes.

) - Spicy

5. While fillets are baking in oven, slice the red and green bell peppers. When ready, remove baking dish from oven and sprinkle the sliced peppers on top of fillets. Bake for 10 minutes.

6. Serve the tilapia fillets over cooked brown and/or wild rice. Pour the bayou sauce over the fillets.

Dessert Recipe

Dark Chocolate-Covered Strawberries (6 servings)

Total time to prepare: 25 minutes

Ingredients:

1 16-ounce dark chocolate bar

6 strawberries

How to prepare:

1. Wash strawberries and allow to completely dry.

2. While the strawberries are drying, melt the dark chocolate bar using a double broiler (two fitted sauce pans the larger of which is filled with water and the smaller of which contains the dark chocolate). Use a low/medium flame to boil water and consistently stir the chocolate with a spoon until the chocolate is completely melted.

3. Once the chocolate is melted, dip a dry strawberry in the pot and place the chocolate-covered strawberry on parchment or wax paper. Allow chocolate covered strawberries to sit until they are completely dry.

DZ Snack

Homemade Popcorn (4-5 servings)

Time to prepare and cook: 10 minutes

Ingredients:

1/3 cup whole grain popcorn kernels

3 tablespoons canola or extra virgin olive oil

1 teaspoon sea salt

How to prepare:

1. Pour canola or extra virgin olive oil in a 3 quart pot (or sauce pan). Allow oil to heat over a low/medium flame.

2. Put a couple of popcorn kernels in the pot. Once the kernels pop, add a 1/3 of a cup of whole grain popcorn kernels and cover the pot with a lid.

3. Once the popping begins, move the pot back and forth across the burner. Once the popping slows, remove the pot from the burner.

4. Pour popcorn into a bowl and add sea salt.

BUC
Optimal Nutrition Chart

The BUC Optimal Nutrition Chart is a weekly 7-day chart that discloses the meals, snacks and drinks that should be consumed to assist in reducing your overall weight, decreasing your waistline, and tearing down the curtain of fat that conceals your six-pack. The chart also will assist in maintaining optimal nutrition which plays a critical role in reducing your risk of cancer, heart disease and other chronic illnesses.

See Chapter Two "Build and Maintain Optimal Health Through Optimal Nutrition" for healthy nutrition strategies, meals, snacks, desserts, and drinks. See Chapter Four "Transitioning to a Lifestyle of Optimal Health" for details on how to make healthy nutrition an integral part of your daily life.

BUC
Optimal Nutrition Chart

	Monday	Tuesday	Wednesday
Pre-Breakfast* Main Course Breakfast	8 oz. Smoothie Add cereal to fruit with skim or low fat milk	8 oz. Smoothie Add hot oatmeal to fruit with or without skim or low fat milk	8 oz. Smoothie Add cereal to fruit with skim or low fat milk
DZ Snack** 1 Water 1 DZ Snack 2 Water 2	Fruit- grapes 16 oz. 1-2 sticks of gum-peppermint 16 oz.	All-natural trail mix 16 oz. Fruit- cherries 16 oz.	Organic or All-natural dried fruit 16 oz. Whole grain granola 16 oz.
Lunch*** sides drink	Grilled chicken breast sandwich Organic black pepper chips Sparkling water- apple	2- 97% Fat Free or "lite" "skinless" beef franks Baked sweet potato fries Acai-Blueberry juice	Chili Whole grain popcorn Sparkling water- guava
DZ Snack 3 Water 3 DZ Snack 4 Water 4	Whole grain granola 16 oz. Dark chocolate bar or pieces 16 oz.	1-2 sticks of gum-spearmint 16 oz Whole grain popcorn 16 oz.	Raw nuts- almond, walnut, pistachio combo 16 oz. Fruit- berries 16 oz.
Dinner**** side dish drink Dessert*****	Grilled salmon Broccoli with wild rice Tart cherry juice Frozen fruit bar	Skinless BBQ chicken breast Black beans with wild-brown rice combo Sparkling water- blackberry 3 Dark chocolate-covered strawberries	Colorful salad with salmon Concord grape juice 2 oz. ice cream sandwich

See Chapter Two "Build and Maintain Optimal Health Through Optimal Nutrition" for detailed description of meals, beverages, desserts, and Danger Zone (DZ) Snacks.

*   Drink Pre-Breakfast smoothie 1-2 hours before Main Course breakfast. Top hot oatmeal with cinnamon.

**   Consume DZ snacks between meals (particularly during times when you feel hungry). For fruit, consume as much as possible. For dark chocolate bar, eat 1 oz. or less. Gum should be sugar-free. For other non-gum DZ snacks, eat one handful.

***   Lunch toppings should include one or a combination of the following: hot peppers, spinach, tomatoes, organic or low fat cheese, organic or all-natural mustard and/or ketchup. Lunch sides should measure one handful. Sweet potato fries should measure approximately 3 oz. (or 12-15 fries). Drinks should be organic or all-natural. Juices should be made of 100% fruit juice with no added sugar.

****   Attempt to eat dinner no later than 7 p.m. Drink at least two 8 oz. glasses of water before dinner. Consume dinner slowly and include a meal halftime.

*****   Following dessert, take an after-meal break: Do not eat any additional food for at least 20 minutes.

Consult your healthcare provider before implementing nutritional or fitness program

BUC
Optimal Nutrition Chart

	Thursday	Friday
Pre-Breakfast* Main Course Breakfast	8 oz. Smoothie Add cereal to fruit with skim or low fat milk	8 oz. Smoothie Add hot oatmeal to fruit with or without skim or low fat milk
DZ Snack** 1 Water 1 DZ Snack 2 Water 2	Raw nuts- pistachios 16 oz. 1-2 sticks of gum- wintergreen 16 oz.	All-natural trail mix 16 oz. Dark chocolate bar or pieces 16 oz.
Lunch*** sides drink	Grilled chicken breast Veggie chips Tart cherry juice	Turkey burger sandwich Organic chipotle chips Cranberry-Raspberry juice
DZ Snack 3 Water 3 DZ Snack 4 Water 4	Dark chocolate bar or pieces 16 oz. Whole grain granola 16 oz.	Organic or All-natural dried fruit 16 oz. Whole grain popcorn 16 oz.
Dinner**** side dish drink	BBQ skinless chicken breast Sweet potato with mixed veggies Sparkling water- blueberry	Skinless tilapia Brown rice with mixed veggies Concord grape juice
Dessert*****	2 Organic fig bars	Frozen fruit bar

See Chapter Two "Build and Maintain Optimal Health Through Optimal Nutrition" for detailed description of meals, beverages, desserts, and Danger Zone (DZ) Snacks.

*   Drink Pre-Breakfast smoothie 1-2 hours before Main Course breakfast. Top hot oatmeal with cinnamon.

**   Consume DZ snacks between meals (particularly during times when you feel hungry). For fruit, consume as much as possible. For dark chocolate bar, eat 1 oz. or less. Gum should be sugar-free. For other non-gum DZ snacks, eat one handful.

***   Lunch toppings should include one or a combination of the following: hot peppers, spinach, tomatoes, organic or low fat cheese, organic or all-natural mustard and/or ketchup. Lunch sides should measure one handful. Sweet potato fries should measure approximately 3 oz. (or 12-15 fries). Drinks should be organic or all-natural. Juices should be made of 100% fruit juice with no added sugar.

****   Attempt to eat dinner no later than 7 p.m. Drink at least two 8 oz. glasses of water before dinner. Consume dinner slowly and include a meal halftime.

*****   Following dessert, take an after-meal break: Do not eat any additional food for at least 20 minutes.

Consult your healthcare provider before implementing nutritional or fitness program

BUC
Optimal Nutrition Chart

	Saturday	Sunday
Pre-Breakfast* Main Course Breakfast	8 oz. Smoothie Add hot oatmeal to fruit with or without skim or low fat milk	8 oz. Smoothie Add cereal to fruit with skim or low fat milk
DZ Snack** 1 Water 1 DZ Snack 2 Water 2	Fruit- berries 16 oz. 1-2 sticks of gum-spearmint 16 oz.	Raw nuts- walnut 16 oz. Whole grain popcorn 16 oz.
Lunch*** sides drink	Lean beef burger Sweet potato fries Cranberry-Blackberry Juice	Roasted turkey breast sandwich Veggie sticks Tart cherry juice
DZ Snack 3 Water 3 DZ Snack 4 Water 4	Raw nuts- almonds 16 oz. Dark chocolate bar or pieces 16 oz.	1-2 sticks of gum- peppermint 16 oz. Fruit- grapes 16 oz.
Dinner**** side dish drink Dessert*****	Colorful salad with chicken breast Acai-blueberry juice 2 oz. ice cream sandwich	Skinless tilapia Brown rice with mixed veggies Sparkling water- orange Dark chocolate bar or pieces

See Chapter Two "Build and Maintain Optimal Health Through Optimal Nutrition" for detailed description of meals, beverages, desserts, and Danger Zone (DZ) Snacks.

*   Drink Pre-Breakfast smoothie 1-2 hours before Main Course breakfast. Top hot oatmeal with cinnamon.

**   Consume DZ snacks between meals (particularly during times when you feel hungry). For fruit, consume as much as possible. For dark chocolate bar, eat 1 oz. or less. Gum should be sugar-free. For other non-gum DZ snacks, eat one handful.

***   Lunch toppings should include one or a combination of the following: hot peppers, spinach, tomatoes, organic or low fat cheese, organic or all-natural mustard and/or ketchup. Lunch sides should measure one handful. Sweet potato fries should measure approximately 3 oz. (or 12-15 fries). Drinks should be organic or all-natural. Juices should be made of 100% fruit juice with no added sugar.

****   Attempt to eat dinner no later than 7 p.m. Drink at least two 8 oz. glasses of water before dinner. Consume dinner slowly and include a meal halftime.

*****   Following dessert, take an after-meal break: Do not eat any additional food for at least 20 minutes.

Consult your healthcare provider before implementing nutritional or fitness program

BUC
Fitness Adventure Chart

The BUC Fitness Adventure Chart will enable you to monitor your Fitness Adventure and compare your progress on a daily, weekly and monthly basis. If you are establishing a fitness plan for the first time or attempting to re-establish (or re-invigorate) a fitness regimen, start by completing a Segment 1 over a 12-week period.

Segment 1 includes warm-up, dynamic stretches, the first four exercises of a Day One, Day Two or Day Three Fitness Adventure (exercises listed below containing an asterisk) and a Home Stretch. Beginning the 13th week, add the next exercise listed on the chart to the Segment 1 exercises. Perform the Segment 1 plus the additional exercise, followed by a Home Stretch, for a 12-week period. Continue this process for each subsequent 12-week period until you are able to complete an entire Day One, Day Two or Day Three Fitness Adventure.

The following is an example of an individual that completed a Day One Fitness Adventure and how the chart should be completed. See Chapter Three "Build and Maintain Optimal Health Through Optimal Fitness" for detailed description of exercises.

Warm-up/Dynamic Stretches*- completed
Interval treadmill run*
   15 minutes +2, max incline-3, max speed-4

V-PAK I*
   Set One- Standard push-ups-4 reps/ Bicycle crunches-4 reps
   Set Two- Close hand push-ups-3 reps/ Bicycle crunches-3 reps
   Set Three-Feet elevated push-ups-2 reps/ Bicycle crunches-2 reps

Tour de Burn*

15 minutes + 2, average speed-2, max speed-4

*V-*PAK II

Set One- Standard chin-ups-4 reps/ 1 ½ Body weight squats-6 reps
Set Two- Pull-ups-3 reps/ 1 ½ Body weigh squats-5 reps
Set Three- Close hand chin-ups-2 reps/ 1 ½ Body weight squats-4 reps

Hanging Knee Raise

Set One- Hanging knee raises-4 reps
Set Two- Hanging knee raise with twist-3 reps

Stand-up Curl

Set One- Supination- 3 reps at 15 pounds
Set Two-Palms Facing In- 2 reps at 20 pounds

Plank

Set One- 20 seconds
Set Two- 10 Seconds

Jump Rope

10 minutes

Home Stretch*- completed

To assure that you are utilizing proper form and technique during the Fitness Adventure, perform exercises in front of a mirror and review the exercise and stretch exhibits every two weeks.

BUC
Week Day
Fitness Adventure Chart
(Example)

Fitness Adventure	Day 1	Day 2
Warm-up and Dynamic Stretches*	√	
Interval treadmill run (minutes/max incline/ max speed)*	15 + 2 / 3/4	
V-PAK I (number of reps)*		
Set One- Standard push-up/Bicycle crunch	4	
Set Two- Close hand push-up/Bicycle crunch	3	
Set Three- Feet elevated push-up/Bicycle crunch	2	
Tour de Burn (minutes/ avg. speed/ max speed)*	15 + 2 / 2/4	
V-PAK II (number of reps)		
Set One- Standard chin-up/1 ½ Body weight squat	4/6	
Set Two- Pull-up/1 ½ Body weight squat	3/5	
Set Three- Close hand chin-up/1 ½ Body weight squat	2/4	
Hanging knee raise (number of reps)		
Set One- Hanging knee raise	4	
Set Two- Hanging knee raise with twist	3	
Stand up curl (number of reps/weight in pounds)**		
Set One- Supination	3/15lbs	
Set Two- Palms Facing In or Up	2/20lbs	
Plank- 2 sets (number of seconds per set)	20/10	
Jump rope (number of minutes)	10	
Home Stretch*	√	

How to use the BUC Fitness Adventure Chart:

Record time, number of reps, etc. for each exercise in appropriate column.

Apply a check mark (√) upon completion of warm-up, dynamic stretches, and Home Stretch.

Monitor progress by comparing results on a daily, weekly and monthly basis.

*   Segment 1

**   For the Stand up curl exercise, perform supination curls for the first set and curls with palms facing in toward the body for the second set of the Day One Fitness Adventure. For the Day Two Fitness Adventure perform supination curls for the first set and curls with palms facing up for the second set.

√   Completed

Consult your healthcare provider before implementing nutritional or fitness program

BUC
Week Day
Fitness Adventure Chart

Fitness Adventure	Day 1	Day 2
Warm-up and Dynamic Stretches*		
Interval treadmill run (minutes/max incline/ max speed)*		
V-PAK I (number of reps)* Set One- Standard push-up/Bicycle crunch Set Two- Close hand push-up/Bicycle crunch Set Three- Feet elevated push-up/Bicycle crunch		
Tour de Burn (minutes/ avg. speed/ max speed)*		
V-PAK II (number of reps) Set One- Standard chin-up/1 ½ Body weight squat Set Two- Pull-up/1 ½ Body weight squat Set Three- Close hand chin-up/1 ½ Body weight squat		
Hanging knee raise (number of reps) Set One- Hanging knee raise Set Two- Hanging knee raise with twist		
Stand up curl (number of reps/weight in pounds)** Set One- Supination Set Two- Palms Facing In or Up		
Plank- 2 sets (number of seconds per set)		
Jump rope (number of minutes)		
Home Stretch*		

How to use the BUC Fitness Adventure Chart:

Record time, number of reps, etc. for each exercise in appropriate column.

Apply a check mark (√) upon completion of warm-up, dynamic stretches, and Home Stretch.

Monitor progress by comparing results on a daily, weekly and monthly basis.

*   Segment 1

**   For the Stand up curl exercise, perform supination curls for the first set and curls with palms facing in toward the body for the second set of the Day One Fitness Adventure. For the Day Two Fitness Adventure perform supination curls for the first set and curls with palms facing up for the second set.

√   Completed

Consult your healthcare provider before implementing nutritional or fitness program

Fitness Adventure	BUC Week End Fitness Adventure Chart
	Day 3
Warm-up and Dynamic Stretches*	
Accelerated interval treadmill run (minutes/max incline/ max speed)*	
V-PAK III (number of reps)* Set One- Stability ball push-up/Stability ball crunch Set Two- Bosu ball push-up/Stability ball crunch with twist Set Three- Reverse stability ball push-up/Stability ball crunch	
Tour de Burn-Deux (minutes/ avg. speed/ max speed)*	
V-PAK IV (number of reps) Set One- Pull-up/1 ½ Bosu body weight squat Set Two- Standard chin-up/1 ½ Bosu body weight squat Set Three- Close hand pull-up/1 ½ Bosu body weight squat	
Bosu oblique crunch- 2 sets (number of reps per set)	
Stand up curl (number of reps/weight in pounds) Set One- Palms Facing In Set Two- Palms Facing Up	
Stability ball plank- 2 sets (number of seconds per set)	
Jump rope (number of minutes)	
Home Stretch*	

How to use the BUC Fitness Adventure Chart:

Record time, number of reps, etc. for each exercise in appropriate column.

Apply a check mark (√) upon completion of warm-up, dynamic stretches, and Home Stretch.

Monitor progress by comparing results on a daily, weekly and monthly basis.

*   Segment 1

√   Completed

Consult your healthcare provider before implementing nutritional or fitness program

BUC
Check the "Extra Luggage"
Nutritional Chart

The Check the "Extra Luggage" nutritional chart represents healthy great tasting room service and restaurant meals I have during business travel to reduce the risk of weight gain. The suggested meals should be used as a guide to maintain optimal nutrition.

I pack various Danger Zone (DZ) snacks to eat between meals. This reduces the risk of overeating during a business lunch or dinner.

BUC
Check the "Extra Luggage"
Nutritional Chart

	Check the "Extra Luggage" 1	Check the "Extra Luggage" 2	Check the "Extra Luggage" 3
Breakfast*	Steel-cut oatmeal with banana & fresh berries Fresh squeezed orange juice	Bran cereal with low fat or skim milk & bananas Fresh squeezed grapefruit juice	Granola with non-fat or Greek yogurt & fresh berries Smoothie
DZ Snack** 1 Water 1 DZ Snack 2 Water 2	Whole grain granola 16 oz. 1-2 sticks of gum- peppermint 16 oz.	Organic or All-natural dried fruit 16 oz. Raw nuts- almonds, walnuts, and pistachios combo 16 oz.	All-natural trail mix 16 oz. 1-2 sticks of gum- peppermint 16 oz.
Lunch*** drink****	Turkey breast sandwich on whole wheat bread or roll Lemonade	Roasted chicken breast on whole wheat pita Iced tea	Spicy chicken tortilla (tomato or spinach) wrap Cranberry juice
DZ Snack 3 Water 3 DZ Snack 4 Water 4	Dark chocolate bar or pieces 16 oz. Raw nuts- almonds, walnuts, and pistachios combo 16 oz.	1-2 sticks of gum- peppermint 16 oz. Veggie chips 16 oz.	Whole grain granola 16 oz. Dark chocolate bar or pieces 16 oz.
Dinner***** Appetizer Main Course drink**** Dessert	Mixed green salad with tomatoes, walnuts, berries and vinaigrette Seafood mixed grilled salmon, tuna, shrimps, scallops & house vinaigrette with side of baby spinach Cranberry juice ¼ of your favorite dessert	Southwestern black bean soup Herb roasted rotisserie chicken with organic baby potatoes and asparagus Lemonade Dark chocolate-covered fruit	Romaine hearts with cucumbers, almonds, berries, and vinaigrette Lemon and herb roasted red snapper with broccoli and brown rice Ice tea Seasonal fruit and berries

* To enhance oatmeal flavor, add a 1/2 tablespoon of cinnamon. You can also add low fat or skim milk.

** Consume DZ snacks between meals (particularly during times when you feel hungry). For a dark chocolate bar, consume 1 ounce or less. Gum should be sugar-free. For other non-gum DZ snacks, consume one handful.

*** For whole wheat rolls, request at least a 1/3 of the dough be removed from the inside of the roll. Sandwich toppings should include mustard, peppers, tomatoes, and/or dark leafy vegetables such as spinach or romaine lettuce.

**** Order unsweetened ice tea or lemonade and flavor yourself.

***** Drink at least two 8 oz. glasses of water before dinner. Consume dinner slowly and include a meal halftime. Following dessert, take an after-meal break: Do not eat any additional food for at least 20 minutes.

Consult your healthcare provider before implementing nutritional or fitness program

BUC
Room Service Workout Chart

The Room Service Workout Chart will enable you to monitor your fitness regimen during business travel. The stretches and exercises can be performed in or within close proximity to your hotel room. Since you will be jumping rope during the workout series, it's beneficial to pack a jump rope when preparing for travel.

The Room Service Workout consists of the following:

Room Service Workout One

Warm-up/Dynamic Stretches
Interval outdoor run
Burpee
Planks
Jump rope
Home Stretch

Room Service Workout Two

Warm-up/Dynamic Stretches
Interval outdoor run
V-PAK V
Bicycle crunches
Jump rope
Home Stretch

Room Service Workout Three

Room Service Workout One
Room Service Workout Two

It is not necessary to perform the Room Service Workout in consecutive order. For example, for one trip, you can perform Workout 2 and the next trip Workout 1. To keep your workout adventurous, add 1 rep to each upper and lower body set (and 1 second to each set of planks) every 4th trip.

The following is an example of a person implementing the Room Service Workout exercises during a series of business trips and how the work out chart should be completed. See detailed description of exercises and number of reps in Chapter Seven "On the Road Again."

BUC
Room Service Workout Chart
(Example)

	Room Service Workout 1	Room Service Workout 2	Room Service Workout 3
Warm-up and Dynamic Stretches	√	√	√
Interval outdoor run (number of minutes)*	15	15	15
Burpee- 2 sets (number of reps per set)	4/3	xx	4/3
Plank- 2 sets (number of seconds per set)	20/10	xx	20/10
V-PAK V (number of reps)	xx		
Set One- Standard push-up/1½ body weight squat	xx	4/6	4/6
Set Two- Close hand push-up/1½ body weight squat	xx	3/5	3/5
Set Three- Feet elevated push-up/1½ body weight squat	xx	2/4	2/4
Bicycle crunch- 2 sets (number of reps per set)	xx	4/3	4/3
Jump rope (number of minutes)	10	10	10
Home Stretch	√	√	√

How to use the BUC Room Service Workout Chart:
Record time, number of reps, etc. for each exercise in appropriate column.
Apply a check mark (√) upon completion of warm-up, dynamic stretches, and Home Stretch.

*   Perform an interval outdoor run modeled after a Day One, Day Two or Day Three interval treadmill run. Use a sports wristwatch to monitor intervals. Use hills (if available) to replicate inclines.

xx   Do not perform this exercise during this Room Service Workout series

√   Completed

Consult your healthcare provider before implementing nutritional or fitness program

BUC
Room Service Workout Chart

	Room Service Workout 1	Room Service Workout 2	Room Service Workout 3
Warm-up and Dynamic Stretches			
Interval outdoor run (number of minutes)*			
Burpee- 2 sets (number of reps per set)		xx	
Plank- 2 sets (number of seconds per set)		xx	
V-PAK V (number of reps)	xx		
Set One- Standard push-up/1½ body weight squat	xx		
Set Two- Close hand push-up/1½ body weight squat	xx		
Set Three- Feet elevated push-up/1½ body weight squat	xx		
Bicycle crunch- 2 sets (number of reps per set)	xx		
Jump rope (number of minutes)			
Home Stretch			

How to use the BUC Room Service Workout Chart:

Record time, number of reps, etc. for each exercise in appropriate column.

Apply a check mark (√) upon completion of warm-up, dynamic stretches, and Home Stretch.

*   Perform an interval outdoor run modeled after a Day One, Day Two or Day Three interval treadmill run. Use a sports wristwatch to monitor intervals. Use hills (if available) to replicate inclines.

xx   Do not perform this exercise during this Room Service Workout series

√   Completed

Consult your healthcare provider before implementing nutritional or fitness program

BUC
Nutrition and Fitness Glossary

A

Ab straps: Cushioned hooped straps attached to metal clips that hook or lock onto a chin up bar. Ab straps are used to perform hanging knee raises and other exercises that tone the abdominal muscles.

Acai: A dark, purple berry produced from the acai palm tree which is native to Central and South America. The acai berry is a potent source of antioxidants which are known to counter the effects of free radicals. Acai is often available in juice form.

Active rest: The 30-to-60 second period between exercise sets in which one is maintaining constant movement to maintain a high calorie burning metabolism.

After Meal Break: Waiting at least 20 minutes before eating any additional food following a meal's dessert to reduce the risk of overeating.

Antioxidants: Molecules that protect the cells of the body by fighting free radicals and may assist in reducing the risk of various health problems such as cancer and heart disease. Sources of antioxidants include black beans, blueberries, raspberries, strawberries, and acai.

Artificial colors: Additives, such as Yellow 5, Yellow 6 and Red 40, used to enhance the color of foods and beverages. Artificial colors have been affiliated with health-related problems ranging from allergic reactions to cancer. Artificial colors are contained in certain cereals, candies, ice creams, and fruit drinks.

Artificial flavors: Additives added to some foods and beverages to enhance flavor. The chemicals used to produce artificial flavors may increase the risk of health-related problems ranging from allergic reactions to cancer. Artificial flavors are contained in certain cereals, ice creams, sodas, and fruit drinks.

B

Beta-carotene: An antioxidant compound that assist in fighting cell damaging free radicals. Beta Carotene provides the orange, red or yellow color in certain foods such as carrots, sweet potatoes and other fruits and vegetables.

Biceps: Muscles located on the front portion of the upper arm, biceps are toned and strengthened through various exercises including push-ups and chin-ups.

Bicycle crunch: Lay on your back with the sole of your right foot on the floor and your left leg extended 2-3 inches off the floor. Place your hands at the sides of your head. Raise your head and shoulders off the floor and contract your abs. While contracting your abs, touch your left knee with your right elbow followed by touching your right knee with your left elbow. Your legs should be moving in a biking motion while your upper torso is moving in a twisting motion. Bicycle Crunches assist in toning Abs.

Big Eating Holidays: Holidays that involve large meal related gatherings that often lead to overeating and weight gain.

Bosu Ball: A ball with a flat bottom and a domed inflatable top. Can be used for various core stability exercises.

Bosu ball push-up: Position the Bosu so that it is lying on the domed, inflatable side. Get into a push-up position. However, place your hands within shoulders width on the flat, rubber side of the Bosu and extend your legs behind you. Your eyes should be facing the Bosu and abs should be contracted. While contracting your abs, lower your body until your elbows are at a 90-degree angle. Then raise your body to the starting position. These push-ups strengthen the core and tone chest, triceps and biceps.

Bosu ball running crunch: Sit on the domed (inflatable) side of the Bosu and lean back until your abs are fully contracted. With legs in mid-air and knees slightly bent, balance yourself on the space between your buttocks and tail bone. From this position, raise your right knee while swinging your left arm, and then raise your left knee while swinging your right arm. During the exercise, your arms and legs should be moving as if you are running. Bosu ball running crunches strengthen the core and tone the abs.

Bosu oblique crunch: Using a Bosu ball, lay on your left side with your hip approximately one inch from the top of the inflatable side of the Bosu. With your hip leaning into the Bosu, cross your ankles, place your hands on the sides of your head, keep your elbows out, and contract your abs. This is the starting position. While contracting your abs, raise your upper torso until your oblique muscles are fully contracted, then lower your upper torso to the starting position. Do the same exercise lying on the right side of your body.

Bosu plyo push-up: Get into a push-up position. However, place your hands on the top center of the Bosu and extend your legs behind you at shoulders width. Lower your body until your elbows are at a 90-degree angle, then explode upward and clap your hands midair. Land with your left hand on the ball and your right hand on the floor. From this position, explode up, clap midair, and land with your right hand on the ball and your left hand on the floor. Bosu plyo push-ups strengthen the core and tone upper body muscles.

Burpee: Stand with your feet at shoulders width, arms at your side, and contract your abs. While contracting your abs, place the palms of your hands on the floor, then kick your feet out behind you. Perform a standard push-up. Then reverse the movement by bringing your knees under your chest with palms of your hands on the floor. Then jump up. Burpees strengthen and tone the entire body.

C

Calcium: A mineral that assist in strengthening bones and teeth. Good sources of calcium include milk, cheese, low- fat yogurt, and leafy green vegetables.

Carboholic: A person who consumes an abundance of refined carbohydrates.

Carbohydrate: A compound contained in certain foods that provides the body with the fuel it needs for physical activity and organ function. Sources of "good" carbohydrates include vegetables, fruit, wholegrain, and beans. Sources of "bad" or refined carbohydrates include white rice, white bread, soft drinks, and other processed foods.

D

Dynamic stretching: Stretching while moving to prepare the muscles of the body for exercise.

E

Empty calories: Calories with little to no nutritional value, included in foods such as candy and soft drinks.

Endorphins: Neurotransmitters in your brain that provide you with a sense of well being or a "feel good" feeling.

Enriching: Occurs when a food manufacturer adds back some of the nutrients removed during the refining/bleaching process. Examples include bleach-enriched flour and bleach-enriched bread.

F

Feet-elevated push-up: Get into a standard push-up position. However, place the toes of your feet on a chair or bench so your legs are elevated. While contracting your abs, lower your body until your elbows are at a 90-degree angle. Then raise your body to the start position. Feet elevated push-ups tone and strengthen chest and arm muscles.

Fiber: A complex carbohydrate not easily digested by the body and, as a result, causes the body to feel full. Good sources of fiber include whole grain, vegetables, fruit, and beans.

Fitness Adventure: A regimen that consists of a variety of cardio, upper body, and lower body exercises.

Fitness Conscious: Consistently being aware of the importance of maintaining healthy nutrition and overall fitness.

Forearm muscles: Located between the wrist and elbow, they are toned and strengthened through various exercises including close-hand pull-ups.

Free radicals: Cell-damaging molecules that have been affiliated with disease and the aging process.

G

Glutes: An abbreviated version of Gluteus maximus which are buttocks muscles.

H

Hanging knee raise: Place each arm in an ab strap (your arms should be positioned at shoulders width) so that your body is supported by your arms and shoulders. Hold the top of the ab straps with your hands and contract your abs. Your body should be hanging from the ab straps with your feet off the floor. While contracting your abs, raise your knees to your chest. Then lower your knees to the starting position. Hanging knee raises tone the abdominal muscles.

Hanging knee raise with twist: Place each arm in an ab strap (your arms should be positioned at shoulders width) so that your body is supported by your arms and shoulders. Hold the top of the ab straps with your hands and contract your abs. Your body should be hanging from the ab straps with your feet off the floor. While contracting your abs, raise your knees to the left, then lower your knees to the starting position, then immediately begin to raise your knees to the right, and then lower your knees to the starting position. Hanging knee raises with twist tones oblique muscles and abs.

Hanging leg raise: Place each arm in an ab strap (your arms should be positioned at shoulders width) so that your body is supported by your arms and shoulders. Hold the top of the ab straps with your hands and contract your abs. Your body should be hanging from the ab straps with your feet off the floor. While contracting your abs, raise your knees to your chest, hold for 1 second, then lower your legs to the starting position then immediately raise your legs to the left until your feet are above your left hand and hold for 1 second. Return to the starting position, then raise your knees to your chest holding the position for 1 second, return to the starting position then immediately raise your legs to the right until your feet are above your right hand and hold for 1 second. Return to the starting position. Hanging leg raises tone ab and oblique muscles.

High fructose corn syrup (HFCS): A manufactured high calorie sweetener and preservative added to various foods or beverages to extend shelf life. HFCS has been affiliated with weight gain and is included in many candies, pastries, sodas, and fruit drinks.

Home Stretch: A series of static stretches following a Fitness Adventure that improves muscle growth, flexibility, range of joint motion, blood circulation, and contributes to muscle relaxation. Each stretch should be held for 20-30 seconds.

Hydrogenated (and Partially Hydrogenated) Oil: Manufactured oil added to various foods to extend food shelf life. This oil can have an adverse effect on heart health. Hydrogenated oils are contained in many baked goods such as cookies and crackers.

I

Intervals: Alternating between slow-and fast-paced speeds during cardio exercises.

Iron: A mineral that assist red blood cells in the delivery of oxygen to the rest of the body and boost the energy level. Good sources of iron include fish, lean meat, poultry, spinach, nuts, and beans.

L

Lattissimus dorsi muscles: Muscles located along the middle/lower portion of the back. "Lats" can be toned and strengthened through various exercises, including chin-ups.

Lavender: A flowering plant in the mint family that has an aroma that has been shown, in some cases, to put the body in a relaxed state.

Lignans: Chemical compounds found in plants that operate as antioxidants. A good source of lignans is flaxseed.

Lycopene: An antioxidant contained in certain foods such as tomatoes.

M

Meal Halftime: Taking a 30-second break halfway through a meal to assist in slowing the pace at which food is consumed to reduce the risk of overeating.

Metabolism: The number of calories the body burns at rest. Aerobic exercises and weight training are ways to increase your body's ability to burn calories.

MSG (Monosodium glutamate): A salt like amino acid that is used to enhance the taste of foods. Several studies have shown that there are certain additives in MSG that may contribute to headaches, chest pain, shortness of breath, nausea, and weight gain. MSG is contained in certain Chinese food, canned vegetables, soups, and processed meats.

O

Oblique muscles: Located along the sides of the abdominal muscles, they can be toned and strengthened through various exercises, including those that involve a twisting motion of the upper torso and Bosu oblique crunches.

Omega-3: "Good" fatty acids that may reduce the risk of heart disease, stroke, and joint point. Good sources include flaxseed, nuts, and fish.

One & Half (1 ½) body weight squat: Place your hands on the sides of your head, position your feet at shoulders width, bend your knees slightly and contract your abs. Keeping your back slightly arched and abs contracted, lower your body until your knees are at a 90-degree angle, then raise your body half way. Then immediately return to the lower position, and then raise body to the starting position (the point where your knees are slightly bent to keep tension on your thighs). The 1 ½ body weight squat exercise tones lower body muscles.

One & Half (1 ½) Bosu body weight squat: Stand on the domed side of the Bosu with feet within shoulders width. Place your hands at the sides of your head and slightly bend your knees. Keeping your back slightly arched and abs contracted, lower your body until your knees are at a 90-degree angle, then raise your body half way, then immediately return to the lower position, then raise your body to the starting position. The 1 ½ Bosu body weight squat exercise strengthens the core and tones lower body muscles. This exercise also can be done on the flat side of the Bosu.

One & Half (1 ½) Bosu body weight squat toss & catch: Stand on the domed side of a Bosu ball with feet within shoulders width. While holding a strength training ball out and in front of your chest, slightly bend your knees and contract your abs. Keeping your back slightly arched and abs contracted, lower your body until your knees are at a 90-degree angle, then raise your body half way while simultaneously tossing and catching the ball (with your finger tips) out and in front of your chest. Then immediately return to the lower position. As you raise your body to the starting position, toss the ball in the air and catch it. The 1 ½ Bosu body weight squat toss and catch exercise strengthens the core and tones the entire body. This exercise also can be done on the flat side of the Bosu.

One & Half (1 ½) Bosu body weight squat with strength training ball: Stand on the domed side of a Bosu ball with feet within shoulders width, slightly bend your knees and contract your abs while holding a strength training ball out and in front of your chest. Keeping your back slightly arched and abs contracted lower your body until your knees are at a 90-degree angle, and then raise your body half way while simultaneously lifting the ball out and in front of your chest. Then immediately return to the lower position with knees at a 90-degree angle. Then immediately raise yourself to the starting position. The 1 ½ Bosu body weight squat with strength training ball exercise strengthens the core and tones the entire body. This exercise also can be done on the flat side of the Bosu.

One & Half (1 ½) chin-up: Using a chin-up bar, get into a chin-up position with your hands slightly within shoulders width, your palms facing your body, and contract your abs. Your body should be hanging with your feet off the floor. While contracting your abs, raise your body half way. Then lower your body to the starting position. Then immediately raise your body until your chin is above the bar. Then lower your body to the starting position. The 1 ½ Chin-up exercise tones and strengths arm and back muscles.

Organic: Food produced in a way that limits the use of synthetic chemicals such as pesticides, insecticides, chemical fertilizers, and chemical herbicides.

P

Plank: Get into a standard push-up position with your eyes facing the floor. However, instead of resting on your hands, rest on your forearms with your elbows (at a 90-degree angle) positioned underneath your shoulders; your forearms should be positioned at shoulders width. Hold this position, while contracting your abs. Planks strengthen the core and tone the abs and shoulder muscles.

Plyo push-up: Get into a standard push-up position with arms at shoulders width and contract your abs. While contracting your abs, lower yourself until your elbows are at a 90-degree angle. Then explode upward raising your torso off the floor and clap your hands mid air. Plyo push-ups tone and strengthen upper body muscles.

Post-Celebration workout: Performed to rev up the body's calorie-burning metabolism following a weight loss celebration meal. The workout consists of a 5-minute moderate speed bike ride on a stationary bike, 5 minutes of jumping rope, and a 5-minute moderate speed treadmill run with little to no rest between each exercise.

Potassium: A mineral that assist in the growth of muscle tissue, prevention of muscle cramps, and may reduce the risk of high blood pressure and stroke. Good sources of potassium include vegetables, beans, and fruit such as bananas.

Pre-Celebration workout: Performed to rev up the body's calorie-burning metabolism prior to a weight loss celebration meal. The workout consists of a 5-minute moderate speed treadmill run, 5 minutes of jumping rope, and a 5-minute moderate speed ride on a stationary bike (or a bike attached to a cycle trainer) with little to no rest between each exercise.

Pull-up: Using a chin up bar, position your hands with palms facing away from your body, hands slightly wider than shoulders width, and contract your abs. Your body should be hanging from the bar with your feet off the floor. While contracting your abs, raise yourself until your chin is above the bar. Then lower yourself to the starting position. Pull-ups tone and strengthen back and arm muscles.

Pull-up-knee-raise: Using a chin up bar, position your hands slightly wider than shoulders width, your palms facing away from your body, and contract your abs. Your body should be hanging with your feet off the floor. While contracting your abs, raise your body until your chin is above the bar. Hold this position and raise your knees toward your chest. Then lower your knees while keeping your chin above the bar. Then lower your body to the starting position. Pull-up-knee raises tone abs and strengthen arm and back muscles.

Pull-up-push-off: Position your hands slightly wider than shoulders width, your palms facing away from your body, and contract your abs. Your body should be hanging with your feet off the floor. While contracting your abs, raise your body until your chin is above the bar. As you slowly lower your body, push your body away from the bar while returning to the starting position. The Pull-up-push-off exercise tones and strengthens arm, back, and chest muscles.

Push-up (standard): Place the palms of your hands on the floor at shoulders width and extend your legs behind you so your body forms a straight line. Your eyes should be facing the floor and your abs should be contracted. While contracting your abs, lower your body until your elbows are at a 90-degree angle. Then raise your body to the start position. Push-ups tone and strengthen the upper body including chest, abdominal, and arm muscles.

R

Raw nuts: Almonds, walnuts, pistachios or other nuts with no added salt, sugar or other ingredient. Nuts are a good source of heart healthy unsaturated fats and Omega-3.

Refining (bleaching): A food process that alters the natural color of certain foods ultimately removing many of the nutrients. Refining/bleaching can deprive the body of fiber-related nutrients such as bran and germ. Refining/bleaching is used to produce foods such as white rice and white bread.

Reps: An abbreviated term for repetition; the number of times a particular exercise is performed.

Reverse stability ball push-up: Get into a standard push-up position. However, position your legs on the stability ball so your shins and tops of your feet are resting along the top of the ball. While contracting your abs, lower your body until your elbows are at a 90-degree angle. Then raise your body to the starting position. Reverse stability ball push-ups strengthen the core and tone chest and arm muscles.

Room Service Workout: Consists mostly of stretches and exercises that can be done in or within close proximity to a hotel room.

Running crunches: Sit on your buttocks and lean back until your abs are fully contracted. With legs in mid-air and knees slightly bent, balance yourself on the space between your buttocks and tail bone. From this position, raise your right knee while swinging your left arm upward, and then raise your left knee while swinging your right arm upward. During the exercise, your arms and legs should be moving as if you are running. Running crunches tone abs.

S

Sea salt: Salt that does not contain additives.

Segment 1: Includes warm-up/dynamic stretches, the first four exercises of a Fitness Adventure and a home stretch.

Set: Consists of a certain number of repetitions or reps.

Six-Pack: A term referring to the 3 sets of abdominal muscles located in the stomach area. A six-pack is developed through a combination of healthy nutrition and exercise.

Split workout: Executing a portion of the Fitness Adventure during a particular time of the day and completing the remaining portion at another time of the day.

Stability (or Swiss) ball: An inflatable ball used for core stability exercises. A stability ball is available in sizes generally ranging from 45 cm to 75 cm.

Stability ball crunch: Sit on the stability ball with legs at shoulders width, knees at a 90-degree angle, and soles of your feet on the floor. Place hands on sides of head and lean back to a position that is slightly greater than a 90- degree angle to keep tension on your abs. While contracting your abs, lean back until your back is on the ball. Then raise your torso to the starting position. Stability ball crunches strengthen the core and tone the abdominal muscles.

Stability ball crunch toss and catch: Sit on a stability ball with legs at shoulders width and knees at a 90-degree angle. While holding a strength training ball above your head, lean back to a position that is slightly greater than a 90 degree angle in order to maintain tension on your abs. While contracting your abs, take 3 seconds to lean back until your back is on the ball. As you raise your upper torso to the starting position, toss the ball above your head and catch it. Tossing and catching the ball increases the difficulty of maintaining balance which strengthens your core and other muscles.

Stability ball crunch with strength training ball: Sit on a stability ball with legs shoulders width apart and knees at a 90-degree angle. While holding a strength training (or medicine) ball above your head, lean back to a position that is slightly greater than a 90-degree angle to maintain tension on your abs. While contracting your abs and holding the strength training ball over head, take 3 seconds to lean back until your back is on the ball and 3 seconds to raise your upper torso to the starting position. Using a strength training ball while performing this exercise makes it more difficult to maintain balance which further strengths your core and other muscles.

Stability ball crunch with twist: Sit on the stability ball with legs at shoulders width, knees at a 90-degree angle, and soles of your feet on the floor. Place hands on sides of head and lean back to a position that is slightly greater than a 90-degree angle. While contracting your abs, take 3 seconds to lean back until your back is on the ball. Then take 3 seconds to raise your upper torso to the right. Then take 3 seconds to lean back again, and then take 3 seconds to raise your upper torso to the left. Stability ball crunches with twist strengthen the core and tone the ab and oblique muscles.

Stability ball plank: Get into a normal plank position, but instead of resting your forearms on the floor, rest your forearms on the top of the stability ball. Contract your abs and keep your body in a straight line. Hold this position. Stability ball planks strengthen the core and tone the abs and shoulder muscles.

Stability ball plank with Bosu: Get into a plank position, but instead of resting your forearms on the floor, rest your forearms on the top of the stability ball while resting your feet on the domed side of Bosu.

Stability ball push-up: Get into a push up position. However, place your hands on the upper sides of the stability ball and extend your legs behind you. Your eyes should be facing the ball and abs should be contracted. While contracting your abs, lower your body until your elbows are at a 90-degree angle. Then raise your body to the starting position. Stability ball push-ups strengthen the core and tone chest and arm muscles.

Stability ball with Bosu push-up: Place your hands on the upper sides of the stability ball. Place your feet on the domed side of a Bosu. While contracting your abs, lower your body until your elbows are at a 90-degree angle. Then raise your body to the starting position. Stability ball with Bosu push-ups strengthen the core and tone upper body muscles.

Stand-up supination curls: Stand with a dumbbell in each hand, legs at shoulders width, chest out, arms close to your torso, palms facing in toward your body, your abs contracted and head in a neutral position facing forward (do not point your chin downward). Before executing a curl, raise each arm to the point in which your elbows are slightly bent and contract your biceps. As you lift the dumbbell in your right hand, rotate your wrist (supination motion) so that your palm is facing upward at the end of the curl. Then reverse the motion as you lower the dumbbell to the starting position. Immediately follow the right hand supination curl with a left hand supination curl. Stand-up supination curls tone and strengthen biceps and forearms.

Strength training (or medicine) ball: A weighted, generally 2-to 25-pound, ball used during various exercises.

T

THE 7: Six ingredients and a form of food processing, at least one of which is used to alter food or beverages in a way that contributes to weight gain and/or a less than healthy diet. The ingredients are high fructose corn syrup, artificial colors, Trans fat, hydrogenated or partially hydrogenated oils, artificial flavors, and MSG. The form of food processing is refining (or bleaching).

Trans Fat: An artificially produced fat used by food manufacturers to extend shelf life. Trans fat has been shown to increase LDL ("bad") cholesterol and lower HDL ("good") cholesterol thus increasing the risk of heart disease. Trans fat is used in the production of various foods such as crackers, cookies, pastries, and some microwavable buttered popcorn.

Triceps: Muscles located along the outside and back of the upper arm. Triceps are toned and strengthened through various exercises, including close-hand push-ups and close-hand pull-ups.

V

Variety Pak (V-PAK): A series of consecutive calorie burning exercises that work different parts of the body. When executing a V-PAK, one part of your body will be allowed to recover while another part is exercising. The maximum active rest between V-PAK exercises is 30 seconds.

Vitamin A: Promotes good vision, healthy skin and strengthens the immune system. Good sources of Vitamin A include cantaloupe, apricots, carrots, sweet potatoes, spinach, broccoli, and peppers.

Vitamin B: Boosts the body's energy level. Fruits and vegetables, such as bananas and broccoli are good sources of vitamin B.

Vitamin C: Boosts the body's immune system. Good sources of Vitamin C include oranges, peaches, strawberries, cantaloupe, mango, peppers, broccoli, tomatoes, and cauliflower.

Vitamin D: Assists in strengthening bones and teeth and reduces the risk of Vitamin D deficiency, which has been associated with osteoporosis, high blood pressure, heart disease, obesity, and certain cancers. Good sources of Vitamin D include milk, eggs, and Wild Sockeye Salmon.

Vitamin E: An antioxidant. Sources of Vitamin E include peaches, papaya, almonds, spinach and other green, leafy vegetables.

Vitamin K: Strengthens bones, normalizes blood clotting, restores damaged cells, and may assist in reducing the risk of osteoporosis. Good sources of Vitamin K include peppers, spinach, and broccoli.

W

Whey Protein: A source of amino acids, available in powder form, which contribute to the growth, repair and maintenance of skin, bone and muscle tissue.

Whole Ground Flaxseed Meal: Flax seed that has been grounded into a powder-like substance. Whole ground flax seed meal is a good source of fiber, lignans and Omega-3.

Wide-arm Bosu push-up: Place the Bosu on the domed side and get into a standard push-up position with hands holding the edges of the ball. While contracting your abs, lower your body until your elbows are at a 90-degree angle. Then raise your body to the starting position. Wide-arm Bosu push-ups strengthen the core and tone upper body muscles.

Workout Ennui: Becoming bored or disinterested with a particular exercise or fitness routine. Covering time monitors during cardio exercises and performing a variety of exercises may reduce the risk of workout ennui.

Acknowledgements

This book would not have been possible without the unending support of family members, friends and colleagues. I like to thank my wife, Sherree, who blesses my body through her nutritional guidance and my spirit with her unconditional love. To my loving children Chanel, Sloan II, and Sterling, whose insatiable energy keep my metabolism revved up and whose growth and development fill my chest with pride. To my "inspirational spotters," Jay Hewlin and Keith Jenkins, for their incessant encouragement which enabled me to exercise my dreams.

A special thanks to J. Michael Falgoust, an accomplished sportswriter, who despite his perpetually busy schedule and endless travel found the time to assist in bringing clarity to my nutrition and fitness principles. Anne Ryan and her team for the creative photographs presented in this book.

I'd also like to thank those who have been a source of inspiration; Colette Luckie, Cecil Luckie, LaTanya Luckie, Sloan J. Harris, Gloria Harris, Sydney Baker, Billy Dexter, Dr. Arthur Mines, Patricia Hewlin, Lauren Fine, Tiffany Dale, Andrew Evans, James "Uncle Brother" Johnson, Darryl Mizel, Singrid Jackson, and the team at Yesterdays Jazz.

Last, but not least, I thank God for granting me the opportunity to share my nutrition and fitness principles. My hope is that this book will assist many in living a healthy abundant life and caring for one of God's greatest creations, the human body. Our bodies truly are "…fearfully and wonderfully made…" Psalm 139:14 (NIV)

This book is dedicated in loving memory of my mother, Sodonia Luckie, the anchor of our family who consistently reminded us that "All things are possible…"

About the Author

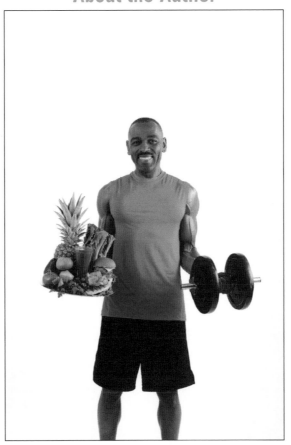

Sloan Joseph Luckie, who is 46 years old, was born in New York City. In 1997, he moved to Chicago where he met his wife, Sherree Elizabeth. Sloan and Sherree have three children, Chanel, 18, Sloan Joseph II, 8 and Sterling William, 5.

Sloan Luckie, a certified public accountant, attained his Bachelor's degree from the University of Hartford and a Masters of Business Administration degree from the NYU Stern School of Business. For more than 12 years, Sloan has been an institutional equity salesman in the brokerage industry.

Sloan is also a financial contributor to the American Cancer Society, American Heart Association, and many other humanitarian programs. His vision is "to reduce the risk of cancer, heart disease, and other chronic illnesses by assisting men and women in developing and maintaining a healthy nutrition and fitness-based lifestyle." He passionately believes a lifestyle built on healthy nutrition and fitness has countless benefits including the ability to:

Reduce the risk of cancer, heart disease and other chronic illnesses

Reduce Stress

Enhance ones quality of life

Improve worker productivity

Significantly reduce health care cost through prevention

Visit **bodyunderconstructiononline.com** for:

Free downloads of BUC Optimal Nutrition and Fitness Adventure Charts

Demos of what, when and how to eat

Fitness Adventure tips and demos

Health-related news and updates

Optimal nutrition meals and recipes

Request for speaking engagement

Much more…

Disclaimer

Sloan J. Luckie is a man with a passion for nutrition and fitness. He believes in and lives a balance of eating nutritious food and exercising. In virtually all respects, he is very much like most of you. That is to say that he is neither a medical doctor nor medical practitioner. He is not a nutritionist, or health specialist. He is not and does not market himself as a personal trainer or physical therapist. He is, however, the average guy (i.e., a man with a full-time job, a home, and children) with an above average, disciplined, lifestyle that has caused him to have a great physique while experiencing optimal health. "Body Under Construction"©, is one of the many ways in which he has chosen to share his experiences in the hope that you will benefit from those experiences.

The book you are holding in your hands or viewing on an electronic device or equipment currently in existence or hereafter created , "Body Under Construction"©, is a product of Body Under Construction, LLC. As such, no part of this book may be reproduced or transferred in any form or by any means, graphic, electronic, or mechanical, including photocopying, recording, taping, or by any information storage retrieval system, or technology, or system, currently in existence or hereinafter created, without the written permission of Body Under Construction, LLC.

As stated above, "Body Under Construction"©, is one of several channels through which Mr. Luckie shares the potential benefits of his lifestyle and the disciplines equated with the same. As such, the book is designed as a general guide, to facilitate your journey toward improved health and fitness. That said, it is important to understand that the accuracy and completeness of information provided herein and opinions stated herein are not guaranteed or warranted to produce any particular results, and the advice and strategies contained herein, may not be suitable for every individual. You are responsible for your health and fitness. Body Under Construction, LLC and Mr. Luckie are not responsible for your health and fitness, and will not be liable for any loss incurred as a consequence of the use and application, directly or indirectly, of any information presented in this book. Matters concerning your health might require medical or professional supervision outside the purpose and scope of this book. Moreover, the ideas, procedures and suggestions provided herein are not intended to replace the advice of licensed medical professionals, licensed nutritionists, licensed physical therapists, or any others within the medical, health, nutrition, fitness, or related fields.

It is recommend that you consult your medical practitioner before adopting any suggestions, particularly if you think you have a condition that might require diagnosis or medical attention. Mr. Luckie and Body Under Construction, LLC do not recommend or endorse any specific medical tests, physicians, products, procedures, or medical opinions. Reliance on any comments or information provided by Mr. Luckie, "Body Under Construction"©, or Body Under Construction, LLC is solely at your own risk. If you are in the United States and are experiencing a medical emergency, please call 911, or call for emergency medical help using the nearest available telephone. If you are outside the US, please call the appropriate number(s) for immediate help.

Body Under Construction, LLC is not responsible for any changes to websites, telephone numbers, books, periodicals, or publications (electronic or otherwise), referenced in the book, "Body Under Construction" ©.

12393932R00107

Made in the USA
Charleston, SC
02 May 2012